THE WAY TO

REDUCE

By
PAUL C. BRAGG, N.D., Ph.D.
LIFE EXTENSION SPECIALIST
and
PATRICIA BRAGG, N.D., Ph.D.
LIFE EXTENSION NUTRITIONIST

Health   *Peace*

Happiness   *Youthfulness*

Love   *Joy*

Praise   *Patience*

Vitality   *Fortitude*

Strength   *Charity*

Faith

JOIN

**The Bragg Crusades for a 100% Healthy, Vigorous,
Strong America and a Better World for All!**

HEALTH SCIENCE
Box 7, Santa Barbara, California 93102 U.S.A.

THE NATURAL
WAY TO
REDUCE

By
PAUL C. BRAGG, N.D., Ph.D.
LIFE EXTENSION SPECIALIST
and
PATRICIA BRAGG, N.D., Ph.D.
LIFE EXTENSION NUTRITIONIST

Copyright © by Health Science. ~ All rights reserved under the International Copyright Union. Printed in the United States of America. No portion of this book may be reproduced or used in any manner without the written permission of the publisher, except by a reviewer who wishes to use brief quotations for a magazine, newspaper, radio or television program. For information address: Health Science, Box 7, Santa Barbara, California, 93102. Telephone (805) 968-1028, FAX (805) 968-1001

- REVISED -
Copyright © Health Science

Eighteenth printing MCMXCII
ISBN: 0-87790-064-7

Published in the United States by
HEALTH SCIENCE - Box 7, Santa Barbara, Calif. 93102, USA

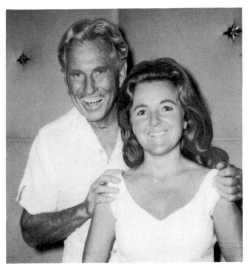

Paul C. Bragg and daughter, Patricia

WHY WE WROTE THIS BOOK

More than 100 million Americans are overweight and the count is mounting— making us the most obese nation in the world! Obesity is now almost an epidemic, reaching into every level and sector of our society. Only a sparse 20% of Americans have some sort of regular exercise program — the rest will suffer the results of sedentary living and lack of exercise which, along with wrong foods, usually brings on cardiovascular diseases and a host of other problems.

Over 52% of Americans living today will die of some form of heart trouble. Being overweight threatens your health by overtaxing every function of your body. Another good reason to normalize your weight: The American Cancer Society's 12-year study led to the shocking fact that obesity increases the risk of a variety of cancers in both women and men. Maybe this is one reason cancer is also almost an epidemic.

In this book, we want to inspire you to start living the Bragg Healthy Heart Lifestyle so you will enjoy a long, vital, healthy life with no problems of obesity and all the other pitfalls that go with it. It is within your power to be the captain of your life for a future filled with radiant health and a trim, fit new you! We know you can achieve your ideal weight, as millions of others have who read the Bragg Health and Fitness Books . . . and are now living the Bragg Healthy Lifestyle for Super Health and Fitness for a Long Happy Life.

We love sharing our Bragg Healthy Lifestyle with you, our dear friends who make our lives so worthwhile and of service spreading health! With blessings of Health, Peace, Joy & Love for You and the World!   - Patricia Bragg

Take time
for **12** things

1   *Take time to Work—*
      it is the price of success.

2   *Take time to Think—*
      it is the source of power.

3   *Take time to Play—*
      it is the secret of youth.

4   *Take time to Read—*
      it is the foundation of knowledge.

5   *Take time to Worship—*
      it is the highway of reverence and washes the
      dust of earth from our eyes.

6   *Take time to Help and Enjoy Friends—*
      it is the source of happiness.

7   *Take time to Love—*
      it is the one sacrament of life.

8   *Take time to Dream—*
      it hitches the soul to the stars.

9   *Take time to Laugh—*
      it is the singing that helps with life's loads.

10   *Take time for Beauty—*
      it is everywhere in nature.

11   *Take time for Health—*
      it is the true wealth and treasure of life.

12   *Take time to Plan—*
      it is the secret of being able to have time to
      take time for the first eleven things.

*From the Bragg home to your home we share our years of health
knowledge—years of living close to God and Nature and what joys of
fruitful, radiant living this produces—this my Father and I share
with you and your loved ones.*

With blessings for Health and Happiness,

Patricia Bragg

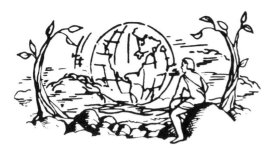

CONTENTS

"To preserve health is a moral and religious duty, for health is the basis for all social virtues. We can no longer be useful when not well."
— Dr. Samuel Johnson, Father of Dictionaries

Contents

When you're dining solo: Sit down, eat slowly and give thanks for your healthy food and your health and then chew your food thoroughly. Remember, your stomach has no teeth! After every third bite, put your fork down and pause and relax. You'll find that the more time you take to enjoy your food by eating slowly, the less food it takes to satisfy you.

THE NATURAL WAY TO REDUCE

If you are reading this book, it is probably because you have more fat on your body that you think is best for you. Good! You've taken the first step toward a healthier, happier life. If you weigh more than you should, you know that being overweight takes its toll on you every minute of every day ... you're probably sluggish and easily tired — and you probably don't feel very good about yourself.

Reduce! Fat is dangerous, fat is unhealthy, fat shortens your life, fat weakens the heart, fat burdens the kidneys. Being fat puts extra strain on your heart, blocks arteries, raises blood pressure, bloats the liver to three times its normal size and finally destroys it. Whether you are mildly overweight (5-10 pounds extra baggage) or deadly overweight (50 or more pounds extra), you must take steps now to rid yourself of that worthless, dangerous fat.

Here's a shocking fact: More than 100 million Americans are obese! It's often because of a lack of exercise and an excessive, careless diet high in salt, fat, sugar and refined foods. In addition, too many people live sedentary lives with long hours in front of the television. What's especially sad is that many of these people are children. We all need sports and exercise to promote a healthy cardiovascular system for a long, healthy life.

This book will show you the dangers that await those who don't get rid of their fat. It will also show you how to change your daily lifestyle ... including eating a better, healthier diet of natural foods and making sure you get a regular dose of invigorating exercise. So you will accomplish two important goals at the same time: losing your fat and transforming your body into a healthy, vigorous, energetic, vibrant person.

If you dedicate yourself to this goal, you will be healthier and happier and you'll look forward to every day. You will also like yourself a lot more when you look in the mirror each morning — and you can bet other people will compliment the new you as well.

1

AVOID THESE PROCESSED, REFINED, HARMFUL FOODS

Once you realize the irreparable harm caused to your body by refined, chemicalized, deficient foods, it is not difficult to eat correctly. Simply eliminate these "killer" foods from your diet...and follow an eating plan which provides the basic, essential nourishment your body needs.

- Refined sugar or refined sugar products such as jams, jellies, preserves, marmalades, yogurts, ice cream, sherberts, Jello, cake, candy, cookies, chewing gum, soft drinks, pies, pastries, tapioca puddings, sugared fruit juices & fruits canned in sugar syrup.

- Salted foods, such as corn chips, salted crackers, salted nuts

- Catsup & mustard w/salt-sugar, Worchestershire sauce, pickles, olives

- White rice & pearled barley   • Fried & greasy foods

- Commercial, highly processed dry cereals such as corn flakes, etc.

- Saturated fats & hydrogenated oils...(heart enemies that clog bloodstream)

- Food which contains palm & cottonseed oil. Products labeled vegetable oil...find out what kind, before you use it.

- Oleo & margarines...(saturated fats & hydrogenated oils)

- Peanut butter that contains hydrogenated, hardened oils

- Coffee, decaffeinated coffee, China black tea & all alcoholic beverages

- Fresh pork & pork products   • Fried, fatty & greasy meats

- Smoked meats, such as ham, bacon & sausage, smoked fish

- Luncheon meats, such as hot dogs, salami, bologna, corned beef, pastrami & any packaged meats containing dangerous sodium nitrate or nitrite

- Dried fruits containing sulphur dioxide - a preservative

- Do not eat chickens that have been injected with stilbestrol, or fed with chicken feed that contains any drug

- Canned soups - read labels for sugar, starch, white, wheat flour & preservatives

- Food that contains benzoate of soda, salt, sugar, cream of tartar...& any additives, drugs or preservatives

- White flour products such as white bread, wheat-white bread, enriched flours, rye bread that has wheat-white flour in it, dumplings, biscuits, buns, gravy, noodles, pancakes, waffles, soda crackers, macaroni, spaghetti, pizza, ravioli, pies, pastries, cakes, cookies , prepared and commercial puddings, and ready-mix bakery products. (Health Stores have a huge variety of 100% whole grain products.)

- Day-old, cooked vegetables & potatoes, & pre-mixed old salads

LET'S LOOK AT FAT REALISTICALLY

All people who carry excess pounds know deep down in their hearts that it's bad for the body to carry this extra burden. They do not have to be nagged and nagged about the seriousness of obesity.

I DO NOT CONDEMN THE FAT PERSON

In my over 50 years of experience as a Physical Conditioner I have met and talked to over-weight people . . . thousands of them. They have been confidential with me and poured out their mental agony of being fat and flabby. They held nothing back from me. I have had men and women break down and cry like babies because they did not have that certain something to reduce and stay reduced. They did not want to be fat. They had read and heard everything about the dangers carrying this excess weight.

They had tried all kinds of "crash" diets, and other diets that promised to reduce them. They went on these diets, lost a few pounds and then for some reason or other went off their diet and gained all the lost weight back again. Over-weight people have told me that they have tried as many as ten to fifteen diets for reducing. Each one of them had failed.

OH NO! NOT ANOTHER BOOK ON HOW TO REDUCE!

When you saw this book your probably made the same remark, "Oh No! Not another book on how to reduce!" I agree with you that the book market is swamped with all kinds of plans for reducing the over-weight person. I know that the magazines and the newspapers of the country are filled with all kinds of diets to try to reduce the over-weight. But practically all these suggested diets are appealing to the weakness of the obese. They tell him he can eat all he wants, will not have to exercise, just follow the simple easy way to make fat melt away without any effort. They all sound so easy.

I wish I could make a promise and say that reducing can be easy. But I am a truthful and sincere person and make no false promises that reducing the natural way is easy. And I will even go further and state that a person who is inclined to add extra pounds to the body will have to maintain some sort of restriction on his diet all the rest of the days of his life.

Fat people do not want to hear such a statement as they feel they do not have the inner strength to be on a sort of reducing diet their entire life-time. But that is the real reason I wrote this book ... I believe there are thousands of fat people who have reached the definite conclusion that it is worth a life-time effort to stay slim and trim. That is the kind of overweight person I am talking to in this book.

NOW LET'S FACE THE FACTS
ABOUT OVERWEIGHT PEOPLE

No two people in the world are exactly alike. Of all the billions of people who have come and gone on this earth, there has never been anyone like you. Your fingerprints, your glandular set-up, your personality are all unique. Because every person is different from everyone else, the way he burns up his food is different, too. We call that metabolism. We burn our foods up at different rates of assimilation. The metabolism of overweight people are inclined to add extra poundage and make flesh out of all the food they eat. That is the reason five blood relatives can sit down at the same dinner table and eat exactly the same amount of the same kinds of foods. Four of them will retain their usual weight, but the fifth person may gain as much as three to five pounds.

So, the first thing to think about before you go on this Natural Way of Reducing is to realize that you cannot eat what everyone else eats and still maintain your normal weight. You are different—you must recognize this fact and eat according to your own personal metabolism. You must study carefully the kinds of foods and the amount of food you eat at each meal. That is why the Natural Way of Reducing is a way of

4

life. It is very much like a person who is born with large feet. Those are the feet that nature equipped him with. Those are the only feet he will ever get. Therefore, he must learn to live with them and adjust himself to them. Now, the same goes for your metabolism. Your body manufactures flesh rapidly, more rapidly than you can burn it up. These are the hard cold facts you must accept about yourself and that is the reason a "crash" diet or a special diet is not going to keep you permanently at normal weight. This is a situation you must face every day of your life. You cannot reduce and then sit back and expect to keep your weight down. It is going to be a life-time job for you. Otherwise you are just going to jump from one new reducing diet to another, always hoping that at last you have found the answer to your overweight problem.

The Natural Way of Reducing will work for everyone. There are no exceptions. For over 50 years I have been using this system on many of the great movie personalities, businessmen, women and statesmen of the world. If you adopt it as your way of life, you too can reduce your weight to normal and then maintain this normal weight. My method works for people who recognize that in their body chemistry there is always a tendency to put on extra pounds. That is the reason it works—it isn't a matter of just taking off the excess weight now carried; it is a matter of taking it off and KEEPING it off.

FIRST STEP TO REDUCING IS IN YOUR MIND

Step one is the beginning of a ten thousand mile journey. Our first step to reducing excess weight and maintaining normal weight is to formulate a mental goal. You cannot enter into a way of life without first deeply desiring to reach certain goals and to always keep these goals in mind.

If you are overweight and would like to reduce, admit you are sick. This is important. Only when you admit that over-eating is an obsession, a compulsion, can you begin to cure yourself.

WHEN YOU ARE HEALTHY AND FIT
YOU ARE HAPPY!

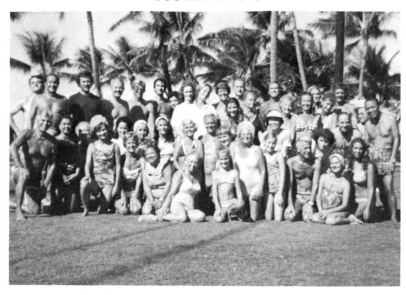

JOIN THE FUN AT THE BRAGG "LONGER LIFE, HEALTH &
HAPPINESS CLUB" WHEN YOU VISIT HAWAII – IT'S FREE!

Paul C. Bragg, daughter Patricia and their wonderful healthy
members of the Bragg "Longer Life, Health and Happiness Club"
exercise daily at the beautiful Fort DeRussy lawn, at the world
famous Waikiki Beach in Honolulu, Hawaii. Membership is free
and open to everyone who wishes to attend any morning – Monday
through Saturday, from 9:00 to 10:30 a.m. for deep breathing,
exercising, meditation, group singing. And on Saturday, after the
class – health lectures on how to live a long, healthy life! The group
averages 75 to 125 per day, according to the seasons.   From
December to March it can go up to 200. When away lecturing, their
dedicated leaders carry on until their return.   Thousands have
visited the club from around the world and then carry the message
of health and fitness to friends and relatives back home. Patricia
extends an invitation to you and your friends to join the club for
wholesome, healthy fellowship . . . when you visit Honolulu, Hawaii.
Be sure also to visit the outer Hawaiian Islands (Maui, Kauai,
Hawaii, Molakai) for a fulfilling, healthy vacation.

---

*To maintain good health the body must be exercised properly (walking, jogging,
running, biking, swimming, deep breathing, good posture, etc.) and nour-
ished wisely (natural foods), so to maintain a normal weight and increase the
good life of radiant health, joy and happiness.*   *- Paul C. Bragg*

Sermons on diet ought to be preached in the churches at least once a week!
— 3 John 2, Pastor G.C. Lichtenberg

If you feel sorry for yourself, good. You have every reason to. But don't let pity turn to hate. Self-hate is the greatest enemy of the overweight person, since it results in pain requiring sedation in the form of food. Only by accepting yourself, whoever and whatever you are, will you be able to change.

Utter hopelessness, the deep down conviction that you can't get well, is your second greatest enemy. It is used again and again as justification for overeating. Why try? Why punish myself? I'm 25 pounds too heavy. Another few pounds is not going to make much difference. The very fact is that your sickness can definitely be cured. But you must be utterly realistic; it's going to be a fight between your mind and your flesh.

EXERCISE YOUR WILL POWER

You must have a powerful desire to want to have normal weight. You have an untapped reservoir of will power, a determination, a will-to-do that can let you achieve anything within reason that you desire. Most people never tap this source of mental energy. It lies dormant and dead most of their lives. You must be aware that it is there and draw upon it daily. It is an unlimited source of mental power. To reduce and stay reduced requires an extra strong determination to carry on this program day after day. You must use your mental power to win over the cravings of the body. In other words, it is mind over matter. Flesh is dumb. There is no intelligence in flesh. The mind must control the flesh at all times. You must recognize that there is a life-long running battle between the mind and the flesh. Flesh is weak—and must be controlled by the mind. Your mind must be strong to restrict the false desires of the flesh. You must be aware that this battle, of the mind and the flesh, will go on until your last day on earth.

Rare Centenarian Couple: I wish everyone would realize it's never too late to turn your life around for the better and maintain a love life!
– Jay and Lila Hoover, 100 and 101 years young of Parma, Idaho

TEMPTATION IS YOUR ENEMY

Man has recognized this demon of false desires for ages. It has been called the Devil and many other names. In the Bible we read the scripture, "Satan, get thee behind me!" We might say, "Temptation, get thee behind me." Because in our modern-day living it is said that all the good things of life are either bad for you or will make you gain weight. Yes, we do live in a world where there is much temptation to eat the wrong foods and drink the wrong drinks. But again I must repeat that if you are going to reduce to your normal weight and maintain that normal weight, you must have firm control over the desires of the flesh. You must be able to say *No* to yourself and you must be able to say *No* to others who tempt you to stray from your program of Natural Reducing.

BUILDING MIND POWER TO CONTROL FLESH

You now know that your greatest enemy is the false cravings of your flesh. The battle lines are now drawn. Our enemy stands before us, daring us to meet his challenge. If we have made up our minds that our mind-power is stronger than the flesh we are ready to enter the battle with confidence. It takes confidence to win battles.

We have two minds: the conscious mind and the subconscious mind. The subconscious mind is the one we must work with to win our battle. Because the subconscious mind is very much like dialing a telephone number: the number we dial is the number we get. We must constantly tell our subconscious mind that we are in complete control of our flesh. The mind sends the messages to the subconscious mind which carries out the orders. When you say, "I am from this day going to control my intake of food," your subconscious mind starts to relay this order to each of the millions of cells of your body. That is the reason we must have two meditations daily. At this time we tell the subconscious mind how the body is to act.

8

The first meditation period must be on arising. It is then ✓
that you meet your subconscious mind and give the orders of
the day. You must use strong affirmations to direct the
subconscious mind. For instance you say, "Today I will so
eat and exercise so that I will lose added pounds." You do not
say your affirmations with a weak will but you put the force
of positive mind-power behind each affirmation. When you
say, "I will!" you mean to follow this declaration with positive actions. That is how you control the desires of human
flesh. Mind over matter. Never let that leave your thoughts.
Your mind is the master. The body is the servant of your
mind. Keep the body in its proper place. It is the servant of
the mind. The mind is the absolute Master of the body. You
must assume this mastership over the body with your mind.
Then your affirmations to the subconscious mind are strong,
positive thoughts which require respect and obedience from
the body.

Over and over repeat, "I am the master of this body. I will
direct its eating and every other action this day that lies
before me." Your affirmations should go like this: "My mind-
power has absolute rule over my body. I am the master. I am
directing the body with intelligence, knowledge and wisdom."

Everything in life is feel and feeling. You must feel the
power of your mind. You must project that power into every
cell of your body ... think positive so you can act positive.
Repeat to yourself ... "I am the absolute master of this
body. Today in these waking hours that lie before me I will
direct the eating, the exercise and the living habits. I have the
power within me, the power given me by my Creator to direct
my body to do as command."

---

*To my mind the greatest mistake a person can make is to remain ignorant
when he is surrounded, every day of his life, by the knowledge he needs to
grow and be healthy and successful. It's all there. We need only to observe,
read, learn ... and apply.*

USE YOUR MIND OR LOSE THE FIGHT

The body must be under constant discipline. You cannot for one moment lose your grip on the body. So say the affirmation and mean it, and follow it up with positive action. Give the orders and the body will be your faithful servant. But the body must know you are the master. The body is always ready to respect the authority of your mind. But if your mind gets lazy ... the body will detect your weakness and will take over instantly. The body has no mind, it is dumb. It wants gratification, it wants thrills, it wants sensations and stimulations. It is the primitive side of your self. It has no control, no safety measure ... eat, drink, and be merry is the code of the body ... live now ... Fill the plate with rich and fattening foods ... drink the drinks that are loaded with calories. Live it up now is all that the body knows ...

But with your God given power of reasoning, you know better than to indulge yourself. You have a conscience. This is the God intelligence within your being. Let your conscience be your guide... not your indulging flesh. Take time each morning to reaffirm faith in yourself. Morning meditation and prayer will give you strength for the day. It means you can design your daily healthy living program each day and the body will carry it out.

MAKE YOUR MIND THE ARCHITECT — BUILDER

After your positive affirmations and after you have given the orders to the subconscious mind for the day's activities, you are ready for visualization ... visualization of the person you want to be. In your mind's eye, which has a great power of imagination, you can picture the kind of person you are building. You see yourself exactly as you want to be ... free of flabby, lardy, ugly fat. You see yourself slim, trim and youthful looking. You see yourself with good muscle and skin tone. Bring that *YOU* into the full focus of your conscious and subconscious mind. Concentrate on the *YOU* that you are building. You must visualize this perfect person you are building. Be able to close your eyes and see this *YOU* standing before you. It must be a crystal clear picture. You see that person; you feel like that person with health, strength, youth and vitality. This is the real you ... do not think of the you that you are now ... the old you is being remodeled.

(continued on page 13)

HEALING HEALTH THERAPIES AND
MASSAGE TECHNIQUES

Explore a few of these wonderful natural methods of healing the body; then choose the technique that's best for your health needs.

F. Mathius Alexander Technique — Lessons intended to end improper use of neuromuscular system and bring body posture back into balance. Eliminates psycho-physical interferences, helps release long-held tension, and aids in re-establishing muscle tone.

Chiropractic — Daniel David Palmer founded chiropractic in 1885 in Davenport, Iowa. From 16 schools now in the U.S., graduates are joining Health Practitioners in all the civilized nations of the world to share their health-healing techniques. Chiropractic is the largest of the non-drug healing professions. Treatment involves soft tissue adjustment and accupressure to free the nervous system of interferences with normal body function. Its concern is the functional integrity of the muscular skeletal system. In addition to manual methods, chiropractors use physical therapy modalities, exercise, health and nutritional guidance.

Feldenkrais Method — Founded by Dr. Moshe Feldenkrais in late 1940s. Lessons lead to improved posture and help create ease and efficiency of movement. A great stress removal method.

Homeopathy — Developed by Dr. Samuel Hahnemann in the 1800s, patients are treated with minute amounts of substances similar to those that cause a particular disease to trigger the body's own defenses. The homeopathic principle is "Like cures like." It is becoming more popular worldwide because it's inexpensive and has minimal side effects.

Naturopathy — Brought to America by Dr. Benedict Lust, M.D., treatment utilizes herbs, diet, fasting, exercise, hydrotherapy, manipulation and sunlight. (Dr. Paul Bragg was a graduate of Dr. Lust's first Naturopathic School in the U.S.) Practitioners reject surgery and drugs except as a last resort.

Osteopathy — The first School of Osteopathy was founded in 1892 by Dr. Andrew Taylor Still, M.D. There are now 15 such colleges in the United States. Treatment involves soft tissue adjustments that free the nervous system from interferences which can cause illness. The complete system of healing by adjustment also includes good nutrition, physical therapies, proper breathing and good posture. Dr. Still's premise was that structure and function of the human body are interdependent and if the structure of the body is altered or abnormal, function is altered and illness results.

(Continued on page 12)

11

Reflexology, or Zone Therapy — Founded by Eunice Ingham, author of "The Story The Feet Can Tell," whose health career was inspired by a Bragg Health Crusade when she was 17. Relieves the body by removing crystalline deposits from meridians (nerve endings) of the feet by using deep pressure massage. A form of Reflexology massage has its early origins in China and is known to have been practiced by Kenyan natives and North American Indian tribes for centuries. Treatment is a firm pressure stroking along the pressure points in the feet by the therapist's fingers.

Reiki — A Japanese form of massage which means "Universal Life Energy." Life energy radiates from the hands of a Reiki therapist. It was discovered in the ancient Sutra manuscripts by Dr. Mikso Usui.

Rolfing — This technique was developed by Ida Rolf in the 1930s in the U.S., and is sometimes called structural processing, postural release or structural dynamics. It is based on the concept that distortions of nominal function of organs and skeletal muscles occur throughout life, and are accentuated by the effects of gravity on the body. Rolfing methods help the individual to achieve balance and improved body posture. Methods involve the use of stretching, deep tissue massage and relaxation techniques to loosen old injuries and break bad movement patterns which cause long-term body stress.

Self Massage — Paul Bragg often said, "You can be your own best masseuse, even if you have only one good hand." Near-miraculous improvements have been achieved by victims of accidents or strokes in bringing life back to afflicted parts of their own bodies by self-massage and even vibrators. Treatments can be day or night, almost continual. Also, self-massage can help achieve relaxation at day's end. Families and friends can exchange massages; it's a wonderful sharing experience. Remember, babies love massages.

Aromatic Massage — It works two ways: The essence (smell) helps the patient relax as does the massage itself, while the massage is used to help absorption of essential natural oils used for centuries to treat numerous complaints. For example, Tiger Balm helps relieve muscle aches. Avoid creams and lotions with mineral oil because it clogs the skin's pores. Almond, olive, peanut and grape seed oil are among the most popular. There are 30-40 aromatics to use derived from herbs and other botanicals. Pure rosemary oil — 6 drops to 6 ounces of almond oil — is a favorite.

(Continued on page 28)

We are not interested in the old you ... only the *NEW* wonderful ... normal weight *YOU*. Burn that picture so deeply in your mind that it becomes a living person. It must never leave your mind's eye. It is a *YOU* that you will be proud of. It will be the *YOU* that will look good dressed or undressed. It is the REAL *YOU*. What the mind conceives and believes it can achieve. Put the new *YOU* under a spot-light, know exactly how that new *YOU* is going to look. Thrill with the feeling of inner joy of your masterpiece. Know that a new *YOU* is in the process of being created. Think of how much pleasure you are going to have with the new *YOU* that you are creating. It will be a thing of beauty ... and a thing of beauty is a joy forever. There is nothing better for a person than a challenge. It gives you a reason for living; it sets the soul on fire. What greater challenge is there than wanting a strong, healthy, youthful body of normal weight. You are working with your most treasured possession, *your body*. Now you are inspired to make it something that will be not only pleasant to look at but it will function with greater efficiency. It will be more alert both physically and mentally. It will be tireless.

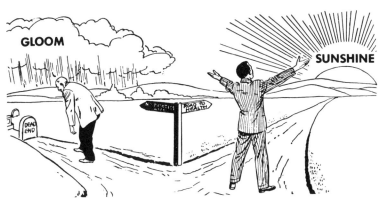

The choice of which road to take is up to the individual. He alone can decide whether he wants to reach a dead end or live a healthy, wholesome, long, active life.

THE HEART AND CIRCULATORY SYSTEM

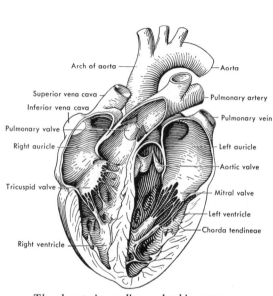

Arch of aorta —

Superior vena cava —
Inferior vena cava —

Pulmonary valve —
Right auricle —

Tricuspid valve —

Right ventricle —

— Aorta

— Pulmonary artery

— Pulmonary vein

— Left auricle

— Aortic valve

— Mitral valve

— Left ventricle

— Chorda tendineae

The heart is really a double pump, each side composed of two chambers, an auricle and a ventricle.

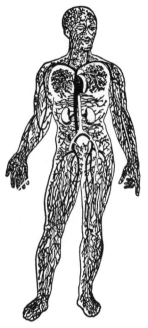

Circulatory system. Showing arteries and veins.

THE PUMP WITH THE BUILT-IN MOTOR

No organ of the body has been paid such flattering court as the heart. It has been romanticized, glamorized, personified, glorified and endowed with emotions, insight, even with intelligence and speech. "The heart has its reasons," we say, and "You must do as your heart tells you."

Primitive tribes ate the heart of an enemy to gain his courage, and not only primitives, but sophisticated ancients believed that one was the seat of the other. The very word courage comes from the Latin word *cor* for heart. Even today we use the two interchangeably, as in the song, from a Broadway success, about what a baseball player needs: "You gotta have heart." Above all, the heart is synonymous with love.

Physicians will admit on occasions that a patient "died of a broken heart," well aware that the heart itself was not medically involved. They mean that the patient lost interest in living; that the mysterious psychic and biological level within him, the will to live that so often pulls an individual back from the brink of death, failed in this instance. The vitality of the organism ebbs away although every ogran may be healthy, including the heart.

Lore and symbol have their logic, and there is a logic to the symbolic aura that glows around the heart. It is the only one of our internal organs that we can actually feel and even hear at its work. We are aware of its pulsations, and by our very mythology of the heart we acknowledge the accuracy with which it reflects our mood. We feel it beating quietly and steadily when we are tranquil, thumping in fright or suspense, pounding strongly when we gather our forces for a dangerous or difficult task. Sometimes it seems to flutter, sometimes to race; sometimes it seems heavy and sometimes light. There are moments when we are sure it leaps into our throat or plummets to the pit of our stomach.

We know that these sensations we ascribe to the heart come from other sources. Obviously, tissues do not change in weight only from emotional provocations. Happy or sad, the adult human heart continues to weigh about a pound. Nor does it change its position in the body. It neither leaps nor drops, but remains safely cushioned between the lungs, resting on their resilience as though on a soft balloon, within the strong spring-like bars of the rib cage.

What does change is its beat, and this changes in both rate and output.

It may jump from a normal 70 or 80 beats per minute to 150 or even 180 in an athlete exerting his supreme effort to win. It is accelerated when we are in the grip of strong emotion. The emotion, as we well know, is in the brain, not the heart, and the heart does not even have any direct nervous system connection with the conscious part of the brain that experiences emotion. It responds, as do all the involuntary mechanisms of the body, to the prompting of the automatic nervous system, whose connections with the emotions are in the hypothalamus of the old, primitive brain. It responds, too, to the adrenalines that pour into the blood stream under the stimulus of excitement.

FAT HINDERS THE WORK OF THE HEART

As you can plainly see, the heart has a tremendous job to do to keep the circulation going over the body; supplying it with nourishment and oxygen.

Now for every square inch of excess fatty tissue, there are 700 miles of small pipe lines that have to feed and nourish this useless fatty tissue. These small pipes are called capillaries. These additional lines put a heavy burden on the heart. That is the reason insurance companies want no part of fat people. They are dangerous risks. The insurance companies know that people carrying excess weight are overworking their hearts and that these people will die long before their time. Many people also die of fatty degeneration of the heart. The heart becomes fat and flabby. The fat, flabby heart just cannot cope with the tremendous burdens that are placed upon it.

The working capacity of the heart is almost incredible. Imagine lifting a thirty-five pound weight, say a packed suitcase, to a height of two feet once every minute; you would be putting out seventy foot-pounds of energy per minute. That is an approximation of what the heart does; it propels more than ten pounds of fluid with enough power to lift it seven feet in the air, every minute of the day. To match it, you would have to lift that thirty-five pound suitcase the same two feet in the air 1,440 times without stopping. This is the heart's ordinary daily work load.

In actual fact, the heart only has to pump its load about as high as you have been lifting your imaginary suitcase the two feet or so, from the heart to head. The additional power is to keep the blood moving along the tortuous pathways of the circulatory system and back again through the veins.

You can prove to yourself how superior the heart muscle is to any ordinary muscle by clenching and unclenching your fist rhythmically in time to a slow count. At what point do the muscles in your hand protest, then ache, and finally quit? You will not be able to make them work again until they have had some rest.

You have been clenching your fist on comparatively unresisting air, but the heart muscle clenches on a rather thick fluid and drives it out into the arteries against the pressure of the blood that already fills them. Try the same experiment with a soft rubber ball or a handful of salt or sugar, and your fist will be attempting something closer to the task of the heart muscle. With the more resistant material to clench on, your hand will probaby tire even sooner than it did the first time. Yet the heart is able to contract a chamber full of fluid, faster than once every second. Furthermore, it does not stop at the count of thirty but goes on pumping day after day, year in and year out, for as long as you live.

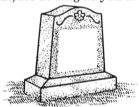

FAT IS THE HEART'S MOST DEADLY ENEMY

As I have told you, every excess pound you carry on your body is a burden to your heart. I have shown you how hard the heart must work to keep you alive. Now, with the excess weight, you pile more work on the heart and that is why the overweight person has the shortest life span.

17

I want you to realize that when you carry excess weight it is not just a matter of appearance; it is a matter of life and death. With each excess pound of weight, you are actually shortening your life. Please concentrate on the seriousness of getting that excess burden off of your heart as soon as possible. I am more interested in keeping you alive than I am of giving you a good personal appearance. Most authorities on weight reduction dwell on how nice you will look when you reach normal weight. I have nothing against a person wanting to look and feel their best. But I am interested in your living out your normal life span. And you are not going to do it if you allow that fat, flabby flesh to remain on your body.

BEING FAT IS A SICKNESS

You are committing slow suicide when you carry excess weight. *YOUR LIFE IS IN DANGER.* While you are alive and carry excess weight you are readily susceptible to many, many diseases that attack sick, flabby flesh and vital organs that are larded with fat. Fat is sick—very sick flesh. Your fat can bring you nothing but trouble and an early ... *GRAVE.* You must get rid of that excess fat and you must keep that fat off your body. Many have won the battle against over-weight and I can help you help yourself to normal weight.

I have students who have carried as much as 200 pounds of fat, flabby, excess flesh on their bodies. I showed them the Natural Way to Reduce and they won their battle. I cannot do it for you. And no one else can. It is your big problem. But with the suggestions given in this book *YOU CAN ATTAIN NORMAL WEIGHT AND KEEP IT.* Don't let anyone tell you that reducing is simple and easy. That is a gross untruth. I will not tell people that the Natural Way to Reduce is easy and that pounds will melt away as some trick diets promise. That is fraudulent. There are no pills, or rather I have no pills, that will melt the weight away. Reducing with drugs, in my opinion, is to sign your own death certificate.

If you have the courage to stick to the Natural Way of Reducing *YOU WILL REDUCE.* It will demand concentration, discipline, courage, positive thinking and positive action.

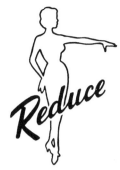

FASTING: NATURE'S GREATEST REDUCER*

Fasting is our first step, and I have placed the hardest step first. Because if you cannot do the hardest part of the reducing program, why waste your time on the program? You are going to have to fast two 24-hour periods every week. And from time to time you are going to have to take a 3-day fast, a 4-day fast and a 7-10 day fast.

And that means you are not going to put any food in your body during that 24-hour fast but ... pure distilled WATER (free of chemicals) ... a full 6 to 8 glasses a day. In cold weather you could have some hot herbal tea or fresh lemon tea using the juice of a fresh lemon. This is often soothing to the stomach. Also you may add a tablespoon of oat bran to your herbal tea if you need better regularity as this is an ideal time to use this wonderful cleanser. It mixes well in herbal tea or water, plus gives you the feeling of fullness in your stomach.

Sure you are going to get hungry. Your flesh is going to cry out for food. But as I told you in the beginning, you are going to rule this flesh of yours with your mind. I mean you are going to be in full control. Let the flesh, which is weak, holler its head off for food. You are going to say, "NO FOOD FOR ME FOR 24 HOURS," and you will win the battle with the flesh.

When you fast you are the complete master of the body. Each time you fast you build more inner strength to carry on your Natural Reducing program. Let me repeat: If you do not have the *Inner Strength* to fast, you will never reduce to your normal weight and maintain that weight. Remember that from the very start of the book I told you that I would be honest with you.

---

* Note: This information is from the Bragg book, "The Miracle of Fasting," a wonderful book that tells all about the incredible health benefits of fasting. See back pages of this book for ordering information.

No man in the world to my knowledge has had the long years I have had in the field of reducing. And I can say without contradiction that you cannot reduce to your normal weight and maintain that weight over the years without fasting. For years I have seen the trick "crash" diets come and go. I have seen people follow these so called "miracle" crash diets. Then a year or so later they had regained all the weight they lost on the tricky diet and had even added a few more pounds of flabby, ugly, sick fat. Please have confidence in my sincerity ... I want to help you accomplish the job of successful reducing, but you must ... *FAST*.

For twenty-five years in California I ran a health resort, and one department was devoted exclusively to reducing. Over-weight people came from all over the world to my reducing institution. Ninety-eight percent of the fat people who came to my health resort learned the Natural Way to Reduce from me. Today, hundreds of those people are following the Natural Way of Reducing to maintain normal weight. They still have to FAST for one to two 24 hours periods a week ... and several times a year they must take 7 to 10 day fasts. As I told you, this is a way of life for the person who is inclined to take on added pounds.

So fast you must. It is rough, it is tough ... but it works! And that is what we are interested in. A program of reducing that will reduce you and keep you reduced. What other over-weight people have done ... *YOU CAN DO*. It just requires a lot of intestinal fortitude, otherwise known as ... *GUTS*.

Any weak-willed, snivelling, flabby weakling can take massages, steam-baths, reducing pills, vibrating machines, 900 calorie liquid drinks per day, rubber clothing, and "crash" diets. They are for the weak-willed. But if you have that deep-down determination to get that sick, deathly, flabby no good ugly fat off of you, you are going to rise to the occasion and find the Inner Strength to fast that deadly fat off your body.

You have to make the decision as to whether you have a backbone or a wishbone. A winner never quits and a loser never wins. You know deep down in your heart that you have the GUTS to fast, and you can get that slobby fat off your body and keep it off. I think every person can rise to any situation, it just takes courage. I know you have it within YOU. We all have it, the creator gave it to all of us, but you have to dig down in yourself and use that courage to save your life. That is what fasting is going to do for you . . . it is going to help you get that fat off your body and keep it off. So let's get started. Let's begin our fasting program and get this reducing job completed so we can enjoy a normal, happy life.

HOW TO FAST FOR 24 HOURS

You can fast from lunch to lunch or from dinner to dinner. Let's say you finish your lunch at 1 P.M. on Monday, then for the next 24 hours you eat nothing and you drink nothing but water. Nothing, no vitamin supplements, no juices, no fruits, no salads. Not anything, just WATER...WATER...WATER. Get that buried deep down in your being. A true fast consists of nothing but pure, distilled water!

When dinner time rolls around you may get some hunger sensations in your stomach. Naturally, the stomach has been accustomed to being fed at this time. This does not mean that you need a dinner, it's merely a reflex action. The stomach has been used to getting food at a certain time, so the reflexes get to work to tell your brain that it is looking for that meal. But we are not going to pay any attention to those reflexes. We are fasting and we are not going to put those calories in our stomach.

Fasting clears away the thousand little things which quickly accumulate and clutter the heart and mind. It cuts through corrosion, renewing our contact with God.

Please be sure to read the Bragg book "The Shocking Truth About Water" for the importance of drinking pure distilled water. See back pages for ordering.

Now something starts to happen, and its wonderful. The body starts to feed on the reserve calories that you have stored in that fat. The body, when fasting, goes after that fat first. This is why the Natural Way of Reducing is so marvelous, you really burn that fat off the body during the fast. Thus, for twenty-four hours you eat nothing. You give the body a physiological rest, and you give the digestive system a rest also.

The liver, the gall bladder and all the other functions you would otherwise use if you had eaten are all given a rest. You have rested them for the first time in your entire life, and with this rest they are going to show their appreciation by doing a wonderful job for you. Your digestive and eliminative system is going to bounce back with greater vitality. You are going to be a better person for giving the body the rest. Sure you may have a headache, sure you may feel a little giddy, you have been used to stimulating yourself with food. Food is a stimulant, but now you are not stimulating the body and it is hollering its head off. But remember I told you that flesh has no sense ... no brains ... flesh is dumb. So why listen to the ravings of a lot of dumb flesh? You have the Brain power to tell the flesh to SHUT UP AND BE QUIET. Talk to that dumb flesh. Tell the stomach that from this day on that you are giving the orders. You are in command. In a few weeks the flesh will recognize you as the master and will be your faithful servant.

WIN OR LOSE IT'S UP TO YOU

As you struggle through the evenings, you are hearing the protesting of your reflexes in the stomach—but you keep yourself busy. Go to a movie, read a good book, visit friends. Drink water to help quiet the appetite. Keep busy and practice thought substitution ... every time your mind wanders to the thought of food, think of something else. GET YOUR MIND OFF FOOD. Don't even talk about food. (You can drink all the water you want during your 24 hour fast, load up if you feel like it.) Drink at least 2 quarts of water per day to help flush out the poisons in the body.

NATURE'S KNOCK OUT PILL

Now, its bed-time and during sleep you fast anyway. This is nature's way of making people fast, for otherwise, people would be eating and snacking for 24 hours around the clock. Some people eat from 7 to 10 times a day. It's breakfast, the coffee break, lunch, the afternoon coffee break, dinner and the snacks before and during the T.V. Show and maybe another snack just before retiring. They have chocolate malts, salted peanuts, pizza pie and ice cream. Some people just never stop feeding their faces all during the waking hours, but nature knocks them cold in sleep so she can get a little physiological rest. The new day begins and this vicious cycle starts all over again. Food ... more food ... cola, drinks, beer, candy, pizza pie, on and on it goes. Yes, man does dig his grave with his teeth or false teeth. Poor weak humans ... eating ... eating ... eating. It is a sickness. And fasting is going to relieve you of your sickness. Fasting is the answer.

You will find that nature certainly will reward you for giving her the rest. So pick two 24 hour periods a week to fast and give your body a chance to burn up fat. You will see the marvelous results, but first you must fast.

DON'T TELL OTHERS THAT YOU ARE FASTING

Reducing the Natural Way should be nobody's business but YOURS. It is your personal problem, so don't tell anyone (EXCEPT THE PERSON WHO PREPARES YOUR FOOD) that you are fasting. Anyone you tell suddenly becomes an expert in reducing and fasting. They will give dire forebodings as to *how* you will damage yourself if you don't stuff food into yourself at regular times. They might even have some hair-raising tales about people who tried to starve themselves thin. Oh my, what tragic tales they can tell you. So, don't open your mouth. This is your personal decision, so don't discuss it. I am the expert with over sixty years of experience in supervision of fasting. You are under my supervision so don't put yourself under the guidance of a knucklehead that knows nothing about fasting. Keep it confidential! Do not discuss it with anyone, for it is none of their business.

DANGEROUS OBESITY BURDENS THE BODY

Please bear in mind that obesity causes sickness! Now we are not talking about the natural fat tissue that is required by the body. Natural fat we carry on various parts of the body acts as a shock absorber. Take, for example, the buttocks— God gave us a padded pedestal to sit on comfortably. This is natural. The heart can pump blood to this part of the anatomy without extra strain. Various organs of the body are cushioned with fat such as the kidneys and liver. This is a part of a healthy body. But we are dealing with excess fat. For instance, if a persons normal weight should, by insurance standards be 150 pounds, but instead weighs 177, that means there are 27 pounds of worthless fat carried on this body. As we have seen, this puts a tremendous burden on a heart that has a hard job to do under normal conditions, without being burdened with 27 extra pounds of worthless toxic fat which is a form of toxic poison. A fat person has a toxin saturated, over- burdened body.

The obese, fat person who comes to us for weight reduction comes to lose weight for the preservation of life itself.

Excess fat weakens your natural resistance to disease and shortens lives. To win the obesity battle you must understand that fat is a toxic poison stored in your body. If you are to win this battle between life and premature death, we must have your complete co-operation. When a student will co-operate, we always warn them at the very beginning of the crisis they will go through when starting on this Natural Reducing and Fasting Program. Their body undergoes a "physiological housecleaning," which was impossible while they were stuffing themselves on foods that originally created fat and toxins in the fluids and tissues of their body. This extra waste is called toxemia, and is a burdensome toxic load of accumulated debris that must be excreted and eliminated. . . if the body is to become healthy and fit!

One can gain a new perspective on food and one's relationship to it by making fasting part of one's way of life—by fasting at regular intervals, preferably one day (24 hours) each week or three consecutive days in each month. — Allan Cott, M.D.

Nature heals through - fasting - every physical problem that it is possible to heal. —Paul C. Bragg

---

Fasting is Cleansing, Purifying and Restful. —Meir Schneider

24

During the 24 hour fasts and other fasts and the natural reducing diet, you may experience quite a bit of turbulence in the body that might bring on some minor headaches, dizziness, weakness, nausea and biliousness. The amount of unpleasant symptoms will depend on how many pounds of excess weight and toxins you carry on the body.

When you take away stimulating foods you will experience a type of "withdrawal symptom" somewhat similar to those suffered by an alcoholic who takes the cure. That is the reason all the many magic, easy reducing plans are doomed from the very beginning. They think that the fat will melt away with no side reactions. Old Mother Nature is a hard mistress and she makes nothing easy for the person who attempts to transgress her laws. You are punished by your dietetic sins. You have to pay a price . . . time & effort to correct and adjust to the Bragg Healthy Lifestyle for life . . . and it's worth it to regain normal weight and super health and fitness again for a long lifetime!

There is absolutely no way to circumvent the laws of Nature. There is no easy road to reducing. If you feel badly at times during the Natural Way of Reducing, this is the law of compensation working. You must pay for what you get in life. As the toxic excess fat is melted away, the disagreeable symptoms then give way to a sense of well-being as the healing process of the body become activated. The power to reduce is within you. When you work with Nature you can accomplish wonders with yourself.

When you fast for 24 hours or 2 to 7 days you are on Mother Nature's operating table cleaning your house that carries you through life! We cannot do anything more than to inspire you to help yourself! The reducing comes from within, and in the end it is you and Nature that does it! If a person is really interested in losing sick, fatty flesh and is really anxious to experience vigorous health (possibly for the first time in his life) . . . you must work 100% with Nature. You must have the courage to make the changes towards super health by cutting down on all excess food intake and by eating smaller portions, by short fasting periods and by having a regular exercise program.

In America, 65% of the population is over-weight. In our opinion, this is the reason so many people die prematurely of heart problems of all kinds, plus a host of other serious ailments.

No goal is reached easily, fasting is a great challenge to the over-weight person. Some over-weight people make feeble attempts at reducing and, because it is difficult, they fall by the wayside and indulge themselves until the overburdened heart collapses and they die before their time.

The Natural Way of Reducing is the only safe, efficient and sure way to reach normal weight. The road is not easy, it is an up-hill climb, but it is worth any real effort you put behind it.

Now we will face the greatest challenge of all, the weekly 24 hour fast. There is nothing complicated about it, you just stop eating for 24 hours and let the body burn fat. Mark the days you are going to fast on your calendar. You are going to fast for two 24 hour periods weekly.

After four weeks of this program you will be ready for a 3 day fast. Do exactly as you did during a 24 hour fast. Eat nothing, but drink all the water you wish. Go about your daily activities as usual. If you get a headache or get some other reaction, just sit down and wait until it passes. You might be one of the lucky ones who fast with a hop, skip and jump without any unusual reactions whatsoever. Many of my students fast for 7 to 10 days and never experience the slightest reaction.

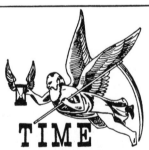

TIME

I have just a little minute,
Only sixty seconds in it,
Just a tiny little minute,
Give account if I abuse it;
Forced upon me; can't refuse it.
Didn't seek it, didn't choose it,
But it's up to me to use it.
I must suffer if I lose it;
But eternity is in it.—Unknown.

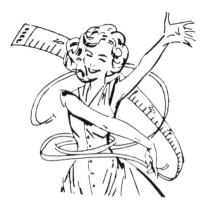

TO BEGIN YOUR NATURAL REDUCING PROGRAM:
THINK TRIM AND SLENDER

Now is the time to put mind over matter, now you must think slender and trimmer. That is, you carry the picture that you have visualized before you at all times! Walk and get the feeling that you are the new reduced You! Do away with sloppy posture; you will walk tall like a trim and fit person, head held high, shoulders up and back, chest out and above. Pull that tummy in, make that tummy touch your backbone (or make it feel that it is touching) and also tighten your seat muscles. Say to yourself over and over "DAY BY DAY I AM GETTING SLIMMER AND TRIMMER." Again repeat...think slim and fit. Visualize yourself as a slim, trim healthy person. Don't tell yourself you are fat any longer! Have no more negative thoughts about excess weight. You are going to visualize yourself slender and trim and filled with super energy for a long, happy, active life.

Over 100 million Americans are overweight. Fat is a killer and a burden on the heart and overall health!

Shocking Facts: *American nationwide health care costs soared to $600 billion in 1991 and this is expected to more than double by the year 2000. This is all the more reason each American should lead a healthy lifestyle to save our economy from this huge medical expense, not to mention the premature death and suffering (physical, mental, emotional and financial).*

Start your daily exercise program today by following the Bragg Health and Fitness Manual. See back pages for ordering.

27

(Continued from page 12)

Shiatsu — It means "finger pressure" in Japanese and is applied with pressure from the fingers, hands, elbows and even knees along the same 12 meridian paths used in acupuncture, which was used for centuries in the Orient to relieve pain, common ills and muscle stress and to aid lymphatic circulation.

Sports Massage — Developed over the years into a sophisticated, important support system for athletes, professional and amateur. Sports massage serves these functions, according to an AMTA brochure: improving circulation and mobility to injured tissue, enabling the athlete to recover more rapidly from myofascial injury, reducing muscle soreness and chronic strain patterns. Soft tissues are freed of trigger points and adhesions, thus contributing toward improvement of peak neuromuscular functioning and athletic performance. It's a preventive approach to injuries that can be suffered during training and it provides a psychological boost to the athlete.

Tragering — Founded by Dr. Milton Trager M.D., who was inspired at age 18 by Paul Bragg to study health. It is an experimental learning method which involves gentle shaking and rocking, suggesting a greater letting go, releasing and lengthening of muscles for body health. Tragering can do miraculous healing where needed in the muscles and entire body.

Water Therapy — Showers are wonderful. First apply olive oil to skin, then hot and cold shower and massage needed areas while under shower. Tub baths are wonderful as well: Apply oil and massage. You can add Epsom salts if your muscles ache or 1 cup of apple cider vinegar. Try dry skin light-brushing — it's wonderful for circulation, toning and healing. Also for variety use a loofah sponge for massaging in the shower and tub.

Swedish Massage — Oldest and most-used massage technique. Deep body massage that soothes, promotes circulation and is also a great way to loosen muscles before and after exercise.

Author's Comment: I have personally sampled all of these techniques, as did my father. Many of the founders were our personal friends. It has made it all the more enjoyable to know how and why they started their health outreach, living lives of service and promoting wellness! In an age where everyone wants health and youthfulness, more and more new styles of massage are becoming popular. My advice to readers: "Seek and find the best for your body, mind, and spirit."

– Patricia Bragg

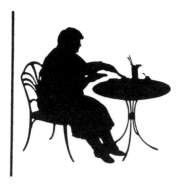

HOW TO EAT DURING THE
NATURAL REDUCING PROGRAM

Before I tell you what to eat and drink, I am going to tell you what *not* to eat. First, we discard salt and anything with salt in it. I want you to regard salt as a poison, which it is, in my opinion. The action of salt is hydration. Salt holds large amounts of liquid and it's stored in fatty tissues, which makes them water-logged – example – swollen legs, ankles, etc. See that your food is prepared without salt. Remember, salt is your enemy! Your fasting program is going to help you eliminate large amounts of salt that now "water-logs" your tissues.

I know you may put up a lot of opposition to this rule, but its difficult to maintain normal weight and use salt or food that has salt added. Now this goes for the rest of your life also. After Reducing the Natural Way, if you go back to eating salt and salty foods, you will gain weight again. There are certain things you must face in life that are hard to adjust to at first. But if you really are serious about staying trim, fit and slender, salt must be removed from your diet forever.

DESSERTS spelled backwards is STRESSED.

Avoid Health-Destroying Habits: *Fat, salt, sugar, white refined flours and chemical preservatives.*

Any type of fish is a healthier choice than the leanest red meat or poultry. Not only is fish low in cholesterol and saturated fat, but it's also high in omega 3 fatty acids, which helps lower cholesterol in the blood.

We know you will ask, "how about social eating, how about my eating in restaurants where the salt has already been added to the food?" Well, we face that problem too. At times we are forced to eat foods that have salt added, but we make them rare exceptions or we fast instead of eating. We know we are often caught up with social eating and dining out at non-health places where salt has been added to the food, but we must try to arrange our lives so we are not forced to eat unhealthy meals. When eating out, we always tell the waiter or waitress that we do not want them to add salt to our food. Salt is bad for the person with normal weight and is extremely bad for the person who is inclined to put on extra pounds.

The first part of a reducing diet eliminates all dairy products including butter, milk (skimmed milk also) and cheese. These foods are almost solid fat and are high in calories. You must have no refined sugars and desserts, no refined breads or sugared cereals, and no soft drinks and no high calorie processed foods!

IDEAL REDUCING SALAD
FOR SUPER HEALTH & LONG LIFE

The best, low calorie diet for the reducer is an abundance of raw, fresh, vegetables of all kinds (organically grown when possible). You must learn to enjoy eating large combination vegetable salads using small amounts of dressings, better yet, just a fresh orange or lemon squeezed over your salad with a dash of Bragg Aminos is delicious and ideal.

Bragg Famous Health Vegetable Salad

2 stalks celery & leaves   1/3 cup red cabbage, chopped
1/2 bellpepper & seeds   1/2 cup green cabbage
1/2 cucumber   1 raw beet, grated
1 carrot, grated   **For Topping:**
2 spring onions & tops   2 tomatoes, diced
1/2 cup alfalfa sprouts   1 avocado, diced

Raw zucchini, yellow squash, sugar peas, mushrooms, broccoli, cauliflower, turnip, may be added for variety. As a salad topping serve in bowl the avocado and tomato mixture, sprinkled with Apple Cider Vinegar and Bragg Aminos. Chop or grate all vegetables fine to medium for variety in size. Mix vegetables thoroughly and serve on a bed of romaine, butter, leaf lettuce or cabbage. Always eat fresh salad at beginning of meal, before serving hot dish. Option— squeeze a fresh lemon or orange over salad as a refreshing, no calorie dressing. Serves 3-4.

Elimination of waste products by fasting increases longevity.
— Alexis Carrel M.D.

Patricia's Health Salad Dressing

1/2 cup olive, soy, canola   *1/4 cup Apple Cider Vinegar*
or flax-seed oil (or blend)   *1/2 tsp raw honey*
3 cloves garlic, crushed   *1/2 tsp Bragg Liquid Aminos*
Optional - *Add various herbs & seasoning as desired:*
Italian herbs, oregano, sweet basil, dill, mustard powder, etc.

Combine all ingredients in jar or blender and mix thoroughly.
Store in refrigerator. For delicious vinegar, add several cloves of
raw garlic and sweet basil to your bottle of Apple Cider Vinegar.

Enjoy Making Healthy Salads

Your body will relish a healthy, large, fresh, raw variety vegetable salad consisting of any of the following: lettuce, sprouts, parsley, celery, radish, broccoli, carrot, cauliflower, beet, cabbage (green & red), tomato, green onion and top, watercress, cucumber and any fresh salad & garden vegetables available. You then can have one or two lightly steamed, baked or stir fry vegetables such as squash, stringbeans, celery, cabbage, spinach, kale, broccoli, cauliflower, corn, carrots, beets, artichokes, mustard greens, lima beans, tomatoes and onions.

You may have moderate amounts of nutritious whole grain pastas, potatoes, beans and legumes. If you are a vegetarian or enjoy delicious vegetarian foods, you may have tofu, soy proteins, soy and nut burgers, and sunflower, pumpkin and sesame seeds, and small amounts of raw nuts and nut butters. If desired you may have as your protein a small portion of organically fed lean meat, poultry, fresh fish and 3-4 fertile, free range eggs per week.

Now how do you put this together in meal form? First, we do not follow the old orthodox way of eating. You must earn your food everyday! Now you can even eat salads, casseroles, fresh fruits or even have the Bragg Health Pep Drink (a meal in itself) for breakfast. . . if you've exercised and earned it first! Remember 6-8 glasses of pure distilled water a day is a must, but not with meals.

Lemon or Orange Fresh Squeeze Squirter is great for reducers . . . roll a lemon or orange on counter to break down the cells for more juice. Poke a small hole in the end. Now you have a super lemon or orange squirter for salads, vegetables, fish dishes, herb teas and with distilled water on fasting days.

Eat a variety of healthy foods; maintain a desirable weight; avoid too much fat, sugar and sodium; eat foods with adequate starch and fiber and it's best to abstain from alcohol and smoking. — Dr. C. Everett Koop, U.S. Surgeon General
Admirer of the Bragg Healthy Lifestyle

Here is a sample day's menu
For the Natural Way of Reducing:

BREAKFAST:

On arising, have a cocktail made of a tablespoon of natural Apple Cider Vinegar with a level teaspoon of honey mixed with distilled water. This cocktail has many nutritional benefits. First it is rich in potassium and most people, especially those who are overweight, are often deficient in this important mineral. Read the Bragg "Apple Cider Vinegar Health System" see back pages for book list. After exercising —walking, stretching, deep breathing, etc. you are ready for some fuel. You may have an apple, banana, pear or orange with either a large dish of lettuce or one hard boiled egg (only 3-4 fertile eggs per week) or a raw salad of your choice, plus a lightly steamed vegetable. We often substitute our Bragg favorite Health "Pep" Drink (see recipe on page 36) for breakfast.

We are strongly opposed to drinking liquids with meals, not just for overweight people but for everyone. So, (now the hard blow) no more beverages of any kind with your meals. You must forever banish coffee, china tea, alcohol, soft drinks and most importantly, salt from your diet. Salt, like caffeine, is a stimulant and are not a part of this Natural Reducing Diet and the Bragg Healthy Lifestyle. (See page 2 for list of foods to avoid.)

SNACKING BETWEEN MEALS ADDS WEIGHT

Snacking between meals will ruin any Natural Reducing Diet. Like stimulants, eating between meals is even more detrimental to the person who is weight-conscious; however, between meals you are allowed to drink as much distilled water as you desire and in moderation fresh vegetable juices (diluted with 1/3 distilled water).

LUNCH:

Start with a health salad — raw grated or sliced carrots, beets, sliced cabbage, green pepper and parsley. Then follow with choice of one or two lightly steamed, wokked or stir-fried vegetables.

For protein, you may have either vegetable or animal protein such as broiled fish, free-range chicken or organically fed beef (a small 6-ounce piece of lean broiled beef, three times weekly) Being vegetarian's we prefer you try the healthy vegetarian proteins from non-animal sources such as tofu, beans, sprouts; raw nuts such as almonds, walnuts and pecans; and raw seeds such as sunflower, pumpkin and sesame seeds.

Healthy Exercise Habit: As I stride along on my daily two-mile brisk walk, I say to myself — often out loud — "Health, Strength, Youth, Vitality, Understanding, Peace, Love, Joy and Salvation for Eternity." It amazes me daily how our wonderful Lord fills my life with all His glorious blessings! — Patricia Bragg

Dinner:

Enjoy mixed sprouts, watercress, celery and tomato for your dinner salad, or mix any three raw delicious vegetables. You may also have one to two lightly steamed or wokked vegetables such as stringbeans, squash and any of the delicious vegetable proteins, or 6 ounces of fresh broiled or sauteed fish (three times weekly). These meals provide sufficient nutrition for the day. Your dinner meal is best not too late and not too much food — after dinner NO T.V. snacks and NO MORE FOOD.

There you have the Bragg Healthy Lifestyle for A Long, Active, Healthy Life . . . the Natural Eating Way to Reduce. You eat five days a week and fast two. So you really eat 15 meals a week, consisting mostly of raw vegetable salads and lightly cooked vegetables. If you are hungry eat plenty of salads, stringbeans, squash or stewed tomatoes. You must learn to fill yourself up on these healthy non-fattening foods.

You must learn to cultivate a taste for delicious raw vegetable salads and healthy cooked vegetables. You must eliminate from your diet the dairy products, refined breads, cookies and cakes and most of all, you must absolutely banish the sugar dessert habit. That is the worst eating habit of all.

Again, it's mind over matter. You must learn to enjoy your healthy, delicious fresh salads and a wide selection of fresh vegetables, fruits and all the other natural, healthy products Health Stores stock.

After you achieve your normal weight . . . you can control your eating with ease. You will be experienced at fasting and if a few extra pounds appear, you can fast them off in a few days!

Restricting the fat in the diet allows more oxygen into our tissue cells, so we will feel more energetic. You have to rid your system of the excess fat to feel best and the most alive, alert, and energetic possible.
— Nathan Pritikin
Who thanked Bragg for inspiring him to a healthy lifestyle.

Fasting cures diseases, dries up bodily humors, puts demons to flight, gets rid of impure thoughts, makes the mind clearer and the heart purer, the body sanctified, and raises man to the throne of God.
— Athenaeus

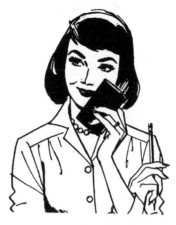

THE DAILY RECORD CHART

If you really mean to Reduce the Natural Way, you have to throw yourself into it whole-heartedly. What is worth doing is worth doing well. You are fighting the demon ... deadly fat. So on your bathroom door, make out a monthly chart. Weigh yourself on your bathroom scale every morning before your vinegar-honey cocktail. Keep a tape measure in the bathroom, measure your waist line every morning and put that down on your chart. There before your eyes you can keep a record of your progress towards the new, slim and trim, healthy *YOU*.

If you are a sincere reducer you will let nothing—absolutely nothing stop you from recording your weight and waist line carefully each day. They are guide lines. Later on, you can have someone take your full measurements. This includes your neck, chest, waist, hips, thighs, and calves. Reducing is a matter of losing pounds and inches off the body.

Weight / Height charts are not for everyone – for we are not all at "ideal" weight levels. Many are heavier than their "ideal" weight because of larger bones, big muscles or both. The pinch-fold test is a more accurate way of determining excessive body fat. Simply pinch the skin on the inside of your upper arm. If the fold between your fingers measures one inch or more in width, you have too much fat.

Healthy Fiber Habit: Make a mixture of two-thirds raw oat bran and one-third psyllium husk powder and use 3-5 tablespoons a day in juices, soups, herbal teas, pep drinks, cereals, muffins, etc., plus ample salads, fresh fruits, vegetables, legumes and 100% whole grains! Fiber helps reduce cholesterol and varicose veins. Fiber helps keep you regular and reduces hemorrhoids and is a natural body weight normalizer.

Thousands of my students all over the world who have used the Natural Way have written me and told me how each reduction, as shown on the scale and the tape measure, has given them that extra something to keep going.

I know I repeat myself many times in this book, but it is done purposely to keep impressing upon you the important points that you must keep in mind in your battle against Killer Fat. Regard fat, every extra pound you carry, as a vicious enemy to your health, well-being and life, and you should fight this deadly enemy with all the power you have within your being.

This is the reason you should not neglect the bathroom chart with your daily weight and the measurement of your waist line.

People find so many excuses to put off doing the really important things in life. You must understand that there is nothing as essential as getting the excess weight off your body ... so *YOUR* body comes first. Business and social obligations and other pressing demands on your time are secondary to your fight for life. Get your values straight. Put first things first—and getting those flabby, sick pounds off your body comes *FIRST*. Mark the days that you fast weekly on the chart and when you go into the longer fasts mark them down. This will give a very accurate picture of your campaign against your excess weight. It can be an inspiration for you to put more effort in the battle.

UNCOMPLICATE YOUR LIVING

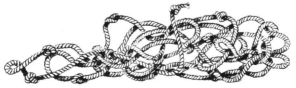

Living is a continual lesson in problem solving, but
the trick is to know where to start. No excuses—
start your Fasting and Reducing Program today.

HEALTHY BEVERAGES
Fresh Juices, Herbal Teas and Pep Drinks

These freshly squeezed vegetable and fruit juices are important to a healthy lifestyle. We feel that it is not wise to drink beverages with your main meals. But if during the day you wish a glass of freshly squeezed orange, grapefruit, vegetable juice, herb tea or try a hot cup of Bragg Liquid Aminos Broth 1/2 tsp - 1 tsp Liquid Aminos in 1 cup hot distilled water. . . They' are ideal pick-me-up beverages.

The Bragg Favorite Juice Cocktail—This drink consists of all raw vegetables (please —organic when possible) which we prepare in our vegetable juicer: Carrots, Celery, Beets, Cabbage, Watercress, Parsley and the purifier Garlic is optional.

The Bragg Favorite Health "Pep" Drink—After our morning exercises often we enjoy this instead of breakfast. Also it's a delicious, nutritious beverage meal anytime . . . even lunch or dinner.

BRAGG HEALTH PEP DRINK
Prepare in blender, add 1 ice cube if desired chilled:

*Juice of 2-3 oranges (fresh) or
  unsweetened pineapple juice
  or 1 glass distilled water
1 tsp raw wheat germ
1/2 tsp brewer's yeast
1 tsp raw oat bran
1/2 tsp psyllium husk powder
1 tsp lecithin granules*

*1/2 tsp Vitamin C powder
1/3 tsp pure pectin powder
1-2 bananas, ripe
1/3 tsp flax seed oil
1 tsp raw honey
1 tbs soy protein powder
1 tsp raw sunflower or
  pumpkin seeds*

Optional: 4 apricots (sun dried, unsulphured). Soak in jar overnight in distilled water or unsweetened pineapple juice. We soak enough to last for several days. Keep refrigerated. In summer you can add fresh fruit in season: peaches, strawberries, berries, apricots, etc. instead of the banana. In winter add apples, oranges, pears or persimmons or try sugar-free, frozen fruits. Serves 1-2.

The nation badly needs to go on a diet. It should do something drastic about excessive, unattractive, life threatening fat. It should get rid of it in the quickest way possible — by fasting. — Allan Cott, M.D.

Fasting is the greatest remedy; the physician within. — Paracelsus

---

Your body has 5 superpumps. Your heart is the masterpump (pumps 2,000 gallons daily), and the other four are your arms and legs that add to it's strength . . . *I spend up to six hours a day waving my arms about . . . if everyone did this, they would stay much healthier!* — Malcolm Sargent, Conductor

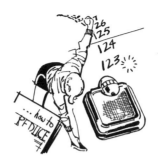

EXERCISE IS AN IMPORTANT PART OF
THE NATURAL WAY TO REDUCE

Fat never remains on an exercised muscle. The two will not mix. Fat is lazy, stupid and degenerate and wants no part of exercise. It can be compared to rats deserting a sinking ship. Fat is flabby and weak and wants no part of exercise whatsoever. Fat is cowardly and just fades away when exercise is applied to it. So with fasting, dieting and exercise . . . flabby, ugly, sick fat is banished. Seems remarkable, doesn't it? But these are the weapons used in the Natural Way of Reducing.

Now I want you to understand what exercise means. It is true that it means at least one half-hour period daily, preferably in the morning. Because if we postpone it, many, many times other responsibilities come and use up the time allotted to exercise. So for your regular exercise period I would make it a point to do it as soon after arising as possible. And don't make a martyr out of yourself. Don't enter it as a slave being driven to a burdensome task. Start your exercise period with a song in your heart. It is natural to want to use your body. It is a sign of youthfulness regardless of your age. The old and senile just sit, the youthful are on the go and active. Just watch children play; they revel in activity, they are never still. I want you to be child-like (not childish). I want you to meet each day of your exercise period joyously and with a song in your heart.

There are only two things in life, feel and feeling. I want you to feel good while you are exercising, knowing that you are keeping the 633 muscles of your body lean, trim and strong. In our daily life, there are always muscles that are being moved. The muscles of digestion are involuntary muscles and work without our command, so does our heart. But we are talking about the larger muscles that we must exercise, the ones that gather fat if not fed and exercised properly.

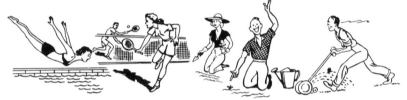

THE BODY IN MOTION

In nature all living things move, and there is infinite diversity in their motion. Some creatures move with marvelous swiftness and control. The dragonfly darts and hovers, the hawk swoops or soars with outspread wings and the small garden snake glides like a shadow out of the path into grassy invisibility. Some forms of life move as imperceptibly as the hour hand on the clock; the plant turns to the sun and its blossoms open and close in such a manner. Slowly or swiftly, they all move. Even the amoeba moves in a leisurely saraband way to embrace its dinner.

Human beings are almost never still. Eyes move, eyelids blink, hands, feet and torso shift even as you sit quietly reading this book. The sleeper changes his position many times during the night. Contrary to the popular notion about sleeping like a log, the most restful sleep is not totally inert. And in our deepest sleep or, conversely, in our most attentive waking moments, when we seem entirely motionless, even then we are kept in constant though scarcely noticeable motion by the heart's steady beating and the muscles of respiration contracting and relaxing as they work the bellows of the lungs.

Most of the thousands of movements that our bodies enact each day are performed without our awareness, and a great many are outside of our voluntary control. Breathing, the propulsion of blood through body and limbs, and of food through the digestive tract are movements powered by muscles that function rhythmically and continuously without our bidding. There are many reflex actions of which we are quite unaware, even as we execute them. There are movements of great complexity, involving the precise timing and co-ordination of many muscles, big and small, that we habitually perform without any notion of how we achieve them. Walking, for instance, or the utterance of meaningful organized sounds that we call speech are movements that once learned, have become automatic. Thus, there is no need for the thinking brain to supervise their performance; it can concentrate on the purpose or meaning of the act rather than the act itself.

A young growing organism, a puppy or a child, is in constant, restless, often explosive through its waking hours and only comparatively quiet in sleep. As we live longer, and substitute a sedentary life for an active one, it is then that the body starts to degenerate and we start putting on the sick, ugly, flabby fat.

TO REST IS TO RUST

As soon as we let the responsibilities of mature adult life dominate us we start to rust. When we were active our muscles and skin had good tone. There was bounce and spring in our bodies. We were lean and trim. Now, most housewives spend their lives doing boresome household duties and most men spend most of their life on their back-sides. Sitting at night clubs, sitting before T.V., sitting in cars, buses, sitting at their desks, sitting at and getting our exercise by proxy watching football, baseball, ballet, swimming meets, tennis matches and all the other sports and pleasures people do sitting.

39

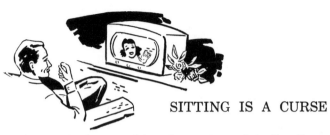

SITTING IS A CURSE

Sitting is the one thing that puts on fat after the consumption of too much food. Inactivity is a curse because it does not burn-up the food you eat. You must burn-up more calories than you eat. Food not burned-up by the body's activity is stored as fat. That is the reason a person puts on excess weight.

I know some people blame their excess weight on faulty functioning of the glands. This may be true of one person in one-hundred thousand but over-weight people like to put all the blame of their excess weight on their glands. No, No, No . . . banish the idea. You are fat because you eat too much and you exercise too little. There are no other excuses. Oh, yes, we hear of the compulsive eater. This is the person who has deep complex emotional problems and who gets release from the tensions of emotional instability by eating and eating and eating. More weak excuses . . . you are a compulsive eater because you have made food your God. But you are not a compulsive eater by nature.

YOU ARE A FOOD DRUNKARD?

Remember, when I started this book I told you I would be honest with you and play the game of reducing with all the cards on the table. I want you to cut out all the alibis and excuses of why you are fat and flabby and face the truth . . . and admit your mistakes. Take a new lease on life and stop excusing yourself for being over-weight. You did it. *YOU*, by eating and inactivity, let yourself get into this condition, and by reversing the process we are going to get every pound of that flabby, fat ugly flesh off your muscles. The muscles are there; they have just been marbled and interwoven with fat. And if we will fast, follow our non-stimulating diet and get active, we can win our battle of the bulge.

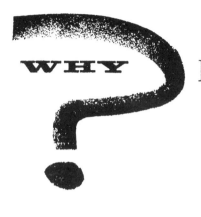

EAT YOUR WAY INTO AN EARLY GRAVE?

FLESH IS DUMB

Flesh has no brain, flesh is by nature lazy. You must motivate flesh into action ... your mind must make those muscles keep active. You must substitute activity for inactivity. We have the most perfect muscular system in the entire animal kingdom. We should develop our muscular skills and develop habits that will keep us active our entire life.

To rest is to rust, and rust is decay. Because you have added years to your life is no reason you should use it as an excuse to be lazy and sedentary. You can have vim, vigor, stamina and spring in every muscle of your body for 100 years or more.

Let the lazy, fat, prematurely old people rot and decay with inactivity. This is not for you! From this day on YOU are going to use every opportunity to use your muscles. You are going to forget elevators and walk up those stairs. And soon the challenge will be fun. As we write this book, my daughter and I are living at the Ilikai

Apartment Hotel in Honolulu; Hawaii is my second home. Our apartment is on the 17th floor. Yes, that's right, the 17th floor and at least once a day I make the round trip, 34 floors of walking, it's a challenge. I am young in heart and neighbors look at me in astonishment, but I enjoy my 17 floors of walking, it's a challenge. I am young in heart and body and I often race the kids who live on my floor up those 17 flights. Yes, Paul Bragg, racing kids up 17 flights of stairs! But I love it. I win a battle every time I make the climb. Now I am not telling you to go out and find a highrise building and see if you can find some kids to race, but you can begin by walking up a few flights to make your muscles work. And do you really have to use that car of yours as much as you do? Of course you don't. We have a car here in Honolulu and I use it only when there are great distances to travel or big loads of fruits and vegetables to purchase and bring home.

Walking is one of my great pleasures in life. On board a ship I walk and run for miles and miles. I revel in breathing the cleanest air in all the world out in mid-ocean. In rain, snow and sunshine I take my daily walk. On the average, I walk 10 miles a day. Here in Honolulu, I walk from my hotel as far down Waikiki Beach as it is possible to walk. My feet are bare, and in the soft sand I feel the 26 bones in each foot being exercised. There is nothing as good for the muscles and nerves of the feet like taking long walks in the sand. I hike up mountains and hills all over the world. A walk sends the circulation racing through my body, opening the arteries and veins so the life's blood will flow fast and wash away the toxic poisons.

Walking is good for the inner man. You can meet your problems without emotion as you walk. I solve all my problems on a long walk, I never try to solve them in my bed. My bed is a place for deep, restful sleep. Take your problems for a long brisk walk and see how fast you can solve them. They cannot be solved when you are lying on your back-side.

Once you get into the habit of walking and using your muscles, you will start to lose fatty spots over the body. Keep this in mind—fat cannot stay on an active muscle.

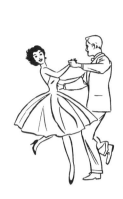
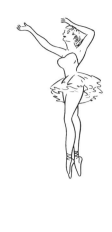

YOU MUST DANCE WHEN FOLLOWING THE
NATURAL WAY OF REDUCING

I am an ardent believer in the kind of activities that bring all the muscles of the body into play. As I have already stated I do not want you to become a slave to exercise. Anything you have to push on yourself becomes burdensome and you just won't keep it up for a lifetime. You have to cultivate a liking and a strong desire to move your 633 muscles.

As I have stated, man is by nature supposed to love physical activity. I meet those kind of people all over the world because I have climbed and I am still climbing the highest mountains in the world. It is one of the thrills of my life to climb a high mountain. I love to swim, and take part in any game or activity that makes my muscles move and work. Exercise is exhilarating.

LEARN TO ENJOY NEW ACTIVITIES

I dance every day of my life. Well, you are going to say, it's impossible for *me* to do. First, you will say I have no one to dance with. Others will say I do not know the new dances, how can I dance? Others will have many other excuses for why they cannot dance.

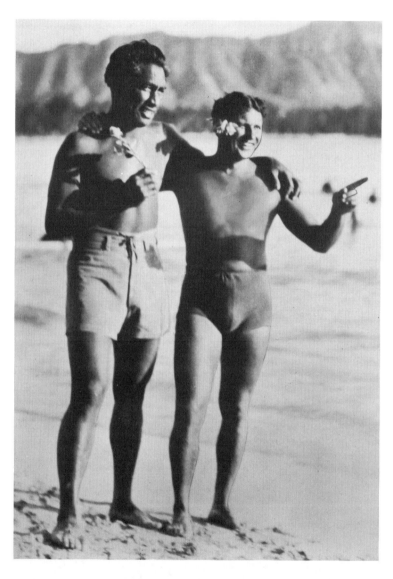

This picture is of Duke Kahanamoku, who was one of the world's greatest athletes in the Olympic Games, and father of modern day surfing. The Duke at one time held every amateur swimming record. Here we see Bragg and the Duke on the beach at Waikiki, a picture taken in the early days of Hawaii'.

Now I will let you in on my deep, dark secret. I dance alone. I turn my radio on morning, noon and night, and I interpret the music just as it makes me feel. Remember what I said, in life there is only feel and feeling. Dancing alone makes me feel wonderful. I make up my own dances as the music pours forth out of the radio. I am not doing an exhibition for anyone. I just dance for the sheer pleasure that it gives me. I always dance bare-footed. What fun I have all alone. I twist, I turn, I circle and jump and I leap. And what natural exercise I get!

EVERYONE SHOULD DANCE

When my own children were very young, we had a victrola and played records just before bed-time. We had a family dance; we put on a gay record and each of us would interpret that record in our own way. Some of the little ones were under five and they made up their own dances by nature or by instinct. It was such a happy time.

I well remember when my father and mother used to visit us from our old home in Virginia. Though they were advanced in years they would take off their shoes and join us in the dance. All my children are still dancing. They danced with their children and now their children's children (my great grandchildren) are dancing. We are four generations of dancers.

Here in Honolulu I have a friend who is one of the most outstanding medical doctors I have known. I have known him for forty years. The good doctor has two dance periods every day. He turns on his radio upon arising and he and his charming wife have the time of their lives with their morning dance. In the evening, just before dinner, radio or the record player is turned on again, the doctor and his wife dance away. Not together, but dancing each in his own way, dancing the way the music makes them feel. The doctor and his wife are in excellent physical condition, they dance their bodies to real fitness.

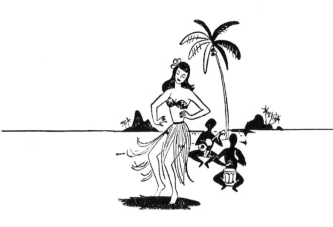

HAWAIIANS LIVE TO DANCE

I call Honolulu my second home and I think it has one of the best climates in the entire world. I speak from experience, as I have circled the world many times. But along with a splendid climate here in Hawaii, nearly everyone dances the Hula, the young and the old, and when there is a party (called a luau), everybody takes their turn dancing. The music plays and away you go, twisting your hips.

Hula dancing is so popular here in Hawaii that they have contests for the children, the teen-agers, the middle-aged and the senior citizens. Some of the best Hula dancers I have seen in these Hawaiian Islands are people in their 60's, 70's and 80's and many nearing the 100 mark. Hula is similar to the dancing I have been telling you about. It is a sort of do-it-yourself project. You wave your arms, roll your hips and swing and sway to the beautiful Hawaiian songs.

I have a small record player that I carry all over the world and I put on a Hula record and get my exercise often in this manner.

I love ball-room dancing too, and I dance whenever I get any chance to. So turn on your radio and dance, dance, dance. These are the activities that keep the muscles free of flabby, ugly fat. Remember what I said, "Fat will not stay on an active muscle."

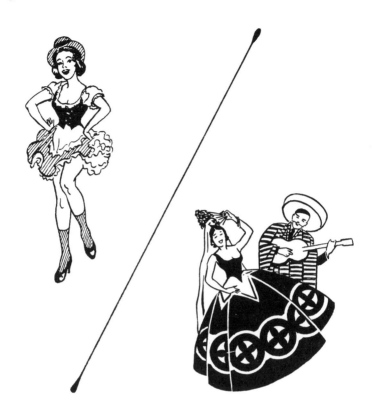

ALL NATIONALITIES LOVE TO DANCE

Look at the Spanish dancers, look at their waist; they have a small waist line. Their bodies are trim and slim and remain so even when they are in their eighties. A few years ago, I was in a rural part of Spain and I attended a dancing contest. The last contest was for people over 70. I was amazed at the grace, the beauty, and most of all the leanness of those dancers. What energy! What vitality! Tears welled in my eyes. I was crying with joy and happiness to see people in the sunset years of their lives doing the Spanish flamenco.

Shame on fat people for allowing their bodies to gob up with ugly fat.

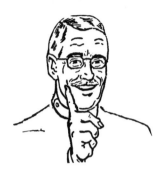

NATURE DESIGNED MAN
TO EXPRESS HIMSELF

Most of the movements our bodies are capable of are shared with other species. The fish swims and the bird flies as automatically as skillfully as a man walks. There are some actions that only a human being can perform. Only man can combine muscle and intelligence and imagination, plan and purpose, to plow and plant the field, to create a museum masterpiece or create and deliver the "Gettysburg Address." And only man trains to perform the most highly co-ordinated forms of bodily motion for their own sake, in the expressive and athletic arts. We applaud this skill in our species every time we clap our hands for a ballerina, star athlete or a circus aerialist.

There is still another kind of motion peculiar to man. Consider the pitcher, the artist of the mound. He bends forward, takes a catcher's signal, makes the mysterious gestures which he believes are essential to his art, and stands motionless for a second. Then he takes a deep breath, draws back, and goes through the series of motions, each one flowing into the next, that constitute the wind-up and the pitch. As the ball leaves his hand, he has completed a perfect demonstration of the beauty of human motion. If the pitch happens to be a third strike and a third out, he may also smile as he walks off the mound, and this is the graceful human touch. Many animals can produce a grimace or a snarl, but only man is equipped with such exquisitely differentiated sets of muscles such as the complex musculature of the face that has no other function than to express and communicate feelings.

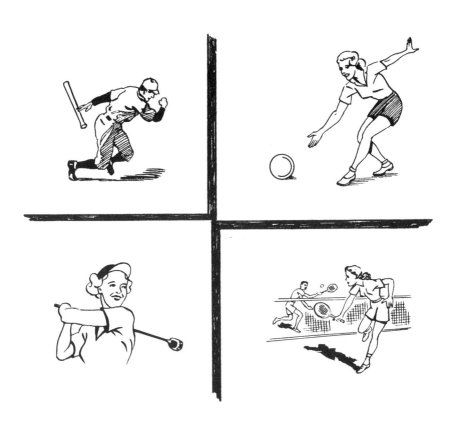

THE GENERATORS OF MOTION

We say of an athlete, "He's in good physical condition," and in this simple statement we embrace a world of physiological meaning. When an athlete is in condition, all the systems and organs of his body are functioning in superb integration. Heart and lungs accelerate smoothly, blood courses at an increased rate and pressure to carry fuel to the muscles and waste products away from them. Kidneys efficiently filter out the waste products and return purified fluids to the body. Eyes are sharp, reflexes quick; brain and nerves sort out perceptions and co-ordinate actions with the economy that we recognize in the simplest motions of a fine performer. No part of the body is inert; the whole splendid organism is committed when the skilled athlete is in top form. And all this integrated functioning is focused on the group of special tissues that generate movement; the muscles.

EXCESS BODY FAT CAUSES HAVOC WITH
HEALTH, SOCIAL, HOME & BUSINESS LIFE

Now when the muscles become marbled and loaded with fat, the muscles become flabby, toxic, lazy and sick. They do not respond well to the directions of the brain. That is the reason fat people are often awkward, clumsy and fall more. They waddle when they walk; the co-ordination between muscles is short-circuited in the toxic sick fat.

Please believe us when we say that our hearts go out in pity to the obese people. We know constant ridicule has a damaging influence on a person's ego. They must be strong to achieve their desired health and fitness goals with daily weigh-ins, keeping a food and exercise log —which keeps you motivated and happy as you progress towards a new, firm, trim you!

Now we realize that every over-weight person is not being laughed at, because they may not be as fat as others. But fat bodies do not move with the grace that lean, fit, trim ones do. Fat is a handicap even if you are 10-15 pounds over your normal weight. The muscles of the over-weight person just do not function as well as they should. Remember, the heart is the strongest muscle in your body, but excess fat can cause it havoc and premature sickness and even death.

WANTED – For Murder of Health & Life

KILLER *Saturated Fats*	CHOKER *Hydrogenated Fats*
CLOGGER *Salt*	DEADEYED *Devitalized Foods*
DOPEY *Caffeine*	HARD *(Inorganic Minerals)Water*
PLUGGER *Frying Pan*	CRAZY *Alcohol*
DEATH-DEALER *Drugs*	SMOKEY *Tobacco*
JERKEY *Turbulent Emotions*	LOAFER *Laziness*
GREASY *Overweight*	HOGGY *Over-Eating*

Walking is Important Part of Reducing Program

No reducing program is complete without a program of systematic walking. The day you start your diet...it's mandatory you start stretching, deep breathing & walking. Begin with a short, brisk walk every day for a week, then each week increase the distance until you walk 2 to 5 miles. For a busy person, brisk walking is the king of erercise and, in conjunction with the diet, is absolutely necessary for successful reducing.

BENEFITS FROM THE JOYS OF FASTING

Fasting is easier than any diet. • Fasting is quickest way to lose weight.

Fasting is adaptable to busy life. • Fasting gives body a physiological rest.
Fasting is used successfully in the treatment of many physical ills.
Fasting can yield weight losses up to 10 pounds or more in first week.
Fasting lowers & normalizes cholesterol & blood pressure levels.
Fasting is a calming experience, often relieving tension and insomnia.
Fasting improves dietary habits. • Fasting increases eating pleasure.
Fasting frequently induces feelings of euphoria, a natural "high".
Fasting is a rejuvenator, slowing the aging process.
Fasting is an energizer, not a debilitator. • Fasting aids elimination process.
Fasting often results in a more vigorous sex life.
Fasting can eliminate or modify smoking, drug, & drinking addictions.
Fasting is a regulator, educating the body to consume food only as needed.
Fasting saves all time spent marketing, preparing & eating.
Fasting rids the body of toxins, giving it an "internal shower" & cleansing.
Fasting does not deprive the body of essential nutrients.
Fasting can be used to uncover the sources of food allergies.
Fasting is used effectively in schizophrenia treatment & other mental ills.
Fasting under proper supervision can be tolerated easily up to 4 weeks.
Fasting does not accumulate appetite; hunger "pangs" disappear in 1-2 days.
Fasting is routine for the animal kingdom.
Fasting has been a commonplace experience since existence for man.
Fasting is a rite in all religions; the Bible alone has 74 references to it.
Fasting under proper conditions is absolutely safe.
Fasting is not starving, it is nature's cure Jesus has given us. - Patricia Bragg
Allan Cott, M.D. "Fasting As A Way Of Life"

Spiritual Reasons Why We Should Fast For
A Healthier, Happier, Longer Walk with the Lord

3 John 2	Deut. 11:7-15, 21	Luke 9:11	Matt. 9:9-15
Gen. 6:3	Gal. 5:13-26	Mark 2:16-20	Neh. 9:1,20-24
I Cor. 7:5	Isaiah 58	Matthew 4:1-4	Psalm 35:13
II Cor. 6	James 5:10-20	Matthew 6:6-18	Romans 16:16-20
Deut. 8:7-8	John 15	Matthew 7	Zechariah 8:19

Dear Health Friend,

This is a gentle reminder of the great benefits from "The Miracle of Fasting" that you will enjoy once you get started on your weekly 24-hour Bragg Fasting Program for Super Health! I fast every Monday and the first 3 days of each month; it's a precious time of body-mind-soul cleansing and renewal. On "fast" days I drink daily 7-9 glasses of pure distilled water or you can have some herb teas or diluted juices. You may add 1 tablespoon of this mixture (2/3 oat bran and 1/3 psyllium husk powder) to these liquids twice a day. Soak mixture two minutes before drinking! It's an extra cleanser and helps normalize weight, cholesterol, blood pressures and helps maintain healthy elimination. Fasting is the oldest, most effective healing method known to man. Fasting offers many Great and Miraculous Blessings from Mother Nature and Jesus.

My father and I wrote the book "Miracle of Fasting" to share with you the health miracles it can perform in your life and it's all so easy-to-do — it's part of the Bragg Healthy Lifestyle.

Patricia Bragg

"The Bragg's work on fasting is one of the great contributions to healing wisdom and the Natural Health Movement in the world today." Gabriel Cousens, M.D., Author "Conscious Eating" and "Spiritual Nutrition".

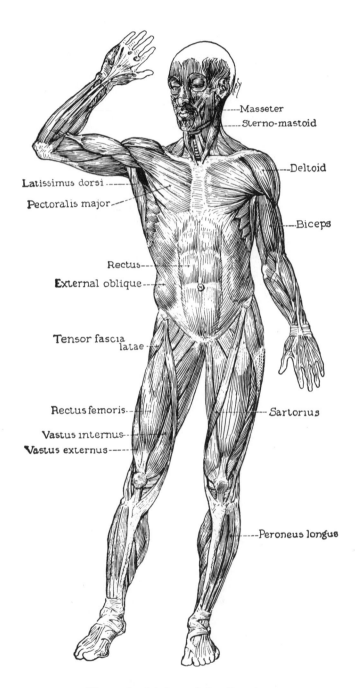

Masseter

Sterno-mastoid

Deltoid

Latissimus dorsi

Pectoralis major

Biceps

Rectus

External oblique

Tensor fascia
latae

Rectus femoris

Sartorius

Vastus internus

Vastus externus

Peroneus longus

The muscles of the human body. Front view.

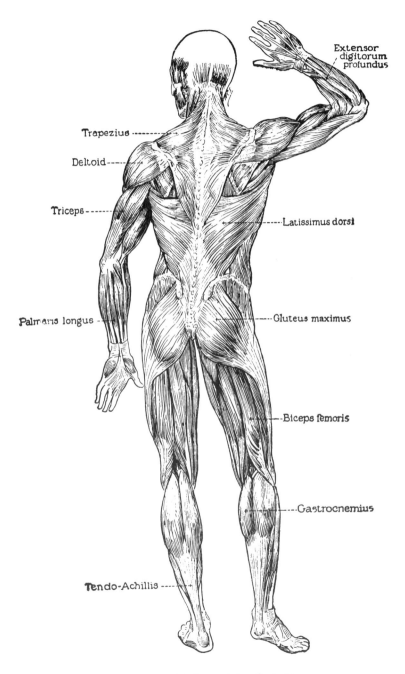

Extensor
digitorum
profundus

Trapezius

Deltoid

Triceps

Latissimus dorsi

Palmaris longus

Gluteus maximus

Biceps femoris

Gastrocnemius

Tendo-Achillis

The muscles of the human body. Back view.

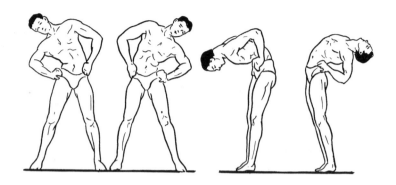

HERE ARE YOUR EXERCISES FOR THE
NATURAL WAY TO REDUCE

Having devoted a lifetime to the study of Physical Culture and Physical Conditioning, I believe I know more exercises than any living expert in this field. I have made it my business in the past 60 years to study the physical culture programs of countries all over the world.

Out of the thousands of exercises, I have selected eleven that I feel an over-weight person should do daily and faithfully along with the diet and the fasting program. These exercises will again restore the muscles back to the natural condition that nature expects them to be in if they are to be of the greatest service to you. Remember, muscles hold you together. Muscles must be firm and fit and have good tone to do their best.

Your exercises should be done in the morning. This is when you have the energy that has been gained during the night. Set your alarm clock and give yourself plenty of time to do these eleven world-famous exercises. Through your fasting and dieting, you will gain more energy to do your exercises vigorously. Remember FLESH IS DUMB. The muscles will not exercise themselves, you have to command the muscles with Mind-Power to do the movements.

Muscles with fat are sick muscles, and you
them to work at your command. You will ;
muscles will ache . . . but you will drive them c
will protest because fatty muscles are lazy mu
will not listen to their cries of "Stop, stop you are hurting
me." Pay them no heed and keep exercising. Remember fat
will not stay on an active muscle and you are going to make
your muscles active.

So away you go every morning. Give yourself from 30 to 45
minutes of exercise. These are the exercises I concentrate my
muscles on. And I have a strong, powerful, fit body. If I can
do them, you CAN AND WILL.

Don't make a big chore out of these exercises. Enter your
exercise with joy in your heart. Get pleasure out of using your
body. Healthy, happy people enjoy this kind of physical
activity. Here they are . . . eleven of the best exercises in the
world. Now they will be yours.

THE ONE, THE ONLY PERFECT EXERCISE— THIS IS IT—THE BEST!

This exercise stretches nearly every one of the six hundred
or more muscles of the body. Stand with your legs apart.
Swing your right arm up and overhead counter-clockwise
across body, then bend from the waist with knees stiff and
touch (or try to touch) your left big toe. You won't do it

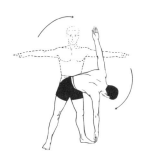

the first time, but stretch down as
far as you can. When your back becomes more supple, you will easily
touch your left big toe. Then whip
arm back overhead, fast and hard,
and bend backwards from the waist.
All this should, of course, be one
continuous movement. Now repeat,
using left arm. Swing left arm up
and overhead, bend and try to touch
the right big toe. While doing this exercise, suck in and blow
out air forcefully, exhaling while touching the toe and inhaling while changing sides. Do the exercise 10 times for each side.

ONE OF THE GREATEST EXERCISES
FOR CIRCULATION

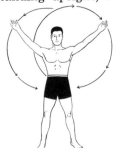

Standing upright, swing both your arms across the front of your body in the opposite direction from each other, up and down in full arm circles. Rhythmically rise on the balls of your feet with each upward swing of the arms, taking regular, full deep breaths, inhaling as you swing the arms up, exhaling as you swing the arms down.

ONE OF THE OLDEST EXERCISES KNOWN
TO MAN AND STILL ONE OF THE BEST

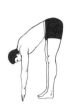

This exercise keeps you supple and flexible . . . stand with toes and heels together, keeping legs together and your knees locked. Raise both hands overhead and stretch them as high as you can. Draw in the diaphragm so it touches your spine (or rather feels that way). Bend at the waist, keeping the knees stiff, and try to touch your toes with your fingertips, but don't strain. You must keep practicing and soon you will touch your toes easily. Exhale as you bend down toward your toes and inhale as you come back to starting position. Do exercise 15 times.

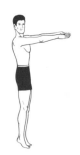

EXERCISE FOR IMPROVING
YOUR BALANCE

Stand up on your toes, with your heels together, your eyes closed, and your arms stretched forward at the shoulders. Stay in this position for 20 seconds without shifting your feet or opening your eyes. Do this exercise 10 times.

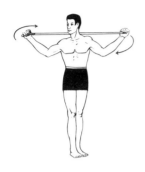

EXERCISES FOR THE SIDE MUSCLES OF THE BODY— THESE MUSCLES ARE KNOWN AS THE BINDING MUSCLES—THEY HELP KEEP YOUR WAIST TRIM, SLIM AND FIRM!

Hold a broomstick behind your neck and shoulders; swing left and right as many times as you can from the waist. Start with ten movements right and left.

STRENGTH-BUILDING EXERCISE FOR HANDS, ARMS, SHOULDERS, BACK, LEGS, ANKLES AND FEET

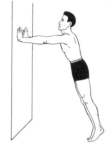

Facing the wall, with your feet placed about thirty or more inches away, lean forward with your hands on the wall, so that the wall is holding you up. Then push up and on your toes and press from toes up through body to hand on the wall. You can also do wall push-ups in this position, where you bend elbows and touch chin to wall.

THE GREATEST EXERCISE FOR STRENGTHENING THE LOWER ABDOMINAL MUSCLES AND THE LOWER SPINE

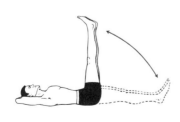

Starting Position: Lie on back with hands clasped behind neck. The Exercise: Holding legs together, raise them to a vertical position, then lower slowly to the floor. Start doing this exercise 5 times, and add more repetitions as your abdomen and spine get strong.

57

TORSO ROTATION FOR STRENGTHENING
WAIST MUSCLES

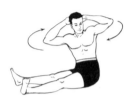

Starting Position: Sit on the floor, with legs extended to the front and both hands clasped behind neck. The Exercise: Twist the upper part of your body to the left as far as you can, then rotate to the right. Do this exercise ten twists on each side.

EXERCISES FOR SLIMMING AND
TRIMMING THE HIPS

Starting Position: Sit with hands on floor beside hips,

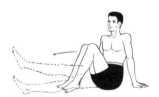

with legs extended. The Exercise: Draw both legs up together until your heels are almost touching your buttocks, then thrust them out to extended position. Do this exercise 10 times — do more as your strength increases.

EXERCISE FOR STRENGTHENING
THIGHS, ABDOMEN AND BACK

Staring Position: Lie on the right side, with left hand on

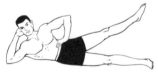

left hip and right hand supporting head. The Exercise: Raise left leg up and down in rapid whipping motion. Do fifteen times on each side.

BACK STRAIGHTENER EXERCISE

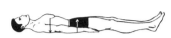

Starting Position: Lie flat on back, with arms at side.
The Exercise: Take a big long full breath, and flatten the lower part of your back to the floor for five seconds, then relax. Repeat 7 times, exhaling fully with release.

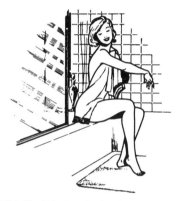

FOLLOW YOUR EXERCISES WITH A COLD BATH AND A COARSE TOWEL FRICTION RUB

There is no tonic which will help to build good skin and muscle tone, as the cold water bath. Cold water is like pure fresh air—it is a natural stimulant. It is the best stimulant to the heart. It is a circulation builder. It stimulates the entire central nervous system. It is a stimulation which is not followed by depression.

------

24 million Americans have osteoporsis which means your bones are porous (holes), more brittle and breakable! This calls for an immediate lifestyle change to 100% health to help eliminate and reverse the problem. How? By improving your diet with more healthy fiber, whole grains, oat bran, fresh fruits, vegetables, sprouts, beans, brown rice, raw seeds, and nuts. Reduce animal proteins for it lowers your calcium levels. Get regular exercise for its revitalizing and promotes healthier bones. Sunshine (vitamin D) in sensible doses is important for healthy bones and makes a big difference to one's health! Not only do you need to get ample minerals from your foods, but take a good, vitamin-mineral supplement daily to insure that you're getting all the necessary nutrients. Researchers state that women over 40 need 1,500 mgs of calcium daily, plus 3 mgs of the trace mineral Boron.

Important—Special Health Insert we want to share with you.

HEALTHY HEART HABITS FOR A LONG, VITAL LIFE

Remember, live foods make live people, and you are what you eat, drink and do so eat a low-fat, low-sugar, high-fiber diet of natural whole grains and starches, sprouts, fresh salad greens, vegetables, fruits, raw seeds, nuts, pure juices and chemical free distilled water.

Earn your food with daily exercise, for regular exercise improves your health, stamina, flexibility, endurance and helps open the cardiovascular system. Only 45 minutes a day can do miracles for your mind and body. You become revitalized with new zest for living.

We are made of tubes: to help keep them clean and open, make a mixture using 2/3 raw oat bran and 1/3 psyllium husk powder and add 2-4 tablespoons daily to juices, pep drinks, herbal teas, soups, hot cereals, foods, etc. Be sure it's wet and expanded for 2 minutes.

Niacin (B-3) helps also to cleanse and open the cardiovascular system. Take regular-released Niacin (100 mg) with one meal daily. Some skin flushing occurs sometimes, nothing to worry about as it shows it's working! After cholesterol level reaches 180 or lower, you can take Niacin once or twice weekly.

Remember, your heart needs a good balance of nutrients, so take a natural vitamin-mineral food supplement with extra vitamin E (mixed Tocopherols), the new Ester-C, Magnesium and Beta Carotene, for these are your heart's super helpers!

Also use this amazing enzyme SOD (super oxide dismutase) for it helps flush out dangerous free radicals that can cause havoc with your cardiovascular pipes and general health. Latest research shows extra benefits . . . promotes longevity, slows aging, fights arthritis and its stiffness, swelling and pain, helps prevent jet lag and exhaustion.

Count your blessings daily while you do your brisk walking and exercises with these affirmations – "health! strength! youth! vitality! peace! laughter! humbleness! energy! understanding! forgiveness! joy! and love for eternity!"– and soon all these qualities will come flooding and bouncing into your life. With blessings of health, peace and love to you, our dear friends and readers.   - Patricia Bragg

---

RECOMMENDED BLOOD CHEMISTRY VALUES

- Total Cholesterol: 180 mg/dl or less, 150 mg/dl or less (optimal)
- Total Cholesterol Childhood Years: 140 mg/dl or less
- HDL Cholesterol: Men: 46 mg/dl or more, Women: 56 mg/dl or more
- HDL Cholesterol Ratio 3.2 or less   •Glucose 80-100 md/dl
- Triglycerides 100 mg/dl or less   •LDL Cholesterol: 120 or less

I know what most of you have been told, "Don't take cold baths—they shock the body!" Don't you believe it! That statement is an untruth. One of the greatest living authorities on Physical Fitness in the world today, Dr. Cureton of the University of Illinois, wholeheartily agrees the cold bath is one of the greatest tonics to the human body. He has spent his life researching on the beneficial effects of the cold bath and strongly urges their use. The colder the better.

I was introduced to cold water bathing in the dead of the winter in Switzerland by the famous Dr. Rollier when I was fighting for my life with T.B. Twice a day, winter and summer, I was given a cold sponge bath followed by a friction towel rub. As I gained new health and strength under Dr. Rollier's supervision, he would give me nude snow baths. The cold water bathing and snow baths gave me a deep, Internal, Physical Fitness ... a fitness unattainable by any other means.

Dr. Rollier told me as I left his great sanitarium, that I must always bathe in cold water to build up my stamina. I have followed his instructions to this very day.

I am Honorary President of the International Society of Polar Bears. This is an organization of men and women the world over who bathe all winter in the coldest weather. I have broken ice and bathed with the Polar Bears in Finland, Sweden, Norway, Germany, Holland, France and even in Moscow, Russia in the intense cold of winter.

I also am a member of three other winter bathing clubs ... The Icebergs of Coney Island, New York ... a happy, healthy, handsome group of winter bathers ... the Boston Brownies of the "L" Street Bathhouse in South Boston, Massachusetts and The Polar Bears at Santa Monica, California.

I can vouch for the supreme health of these cold water bathers. There are very few overweight people in these organizations. And I can say they have the best skin and muscle tone of any people I have met in the entire world.

Now toss out the negative warnings of the flabby, sickly, shivering weaklings. After you finish your exercises learn to delight in the joys and beneficial healthy results of cold water bathing. Certainly it will require some courage to start but once you get the habit of cold water bathing it becomes one of the greatest events in your life.

Start with lukewarm water at the beginning and gradually make the water colder and colder and COLDER.

Get yourself a really good stiff bath-brush and go to work on your skin. Scrub until it is pink. After your cold bath take a big towel (PURCHASE SEVERAL LARGE THICK COARSE TOWELS) and give yourself a rub down with that coarse towel until you are a brilliant red. This is one of the greatest aids to skin and muscle tone; but you must rub, rub, RUB.

Yes, it will be difficult at first. Don't let this important part of the reducing program pass you by. As you carry on your Natural Way to Reduce and eat your non-stimulating diet and do your two 24 hour periods of weekly fasting, fat will melt away and the real *YOU* will reveal itself. You will be mighty proud of that new body of yours. Then the cold water will thrill you no end.

I have often been on ships where I have been the only swimmer in the pool because the weather and water in the swimming pool was cool. I have fun swimming in cold water. And I want you to learn to have fun with your cold baths.

As the teenager's say "Don't chicken out". Grit your teeth and plunge into that cold bath . . . soon you will feel the blood rushing through your body and then to your great surprise you will look at your skin and see something that will really warm your heart.

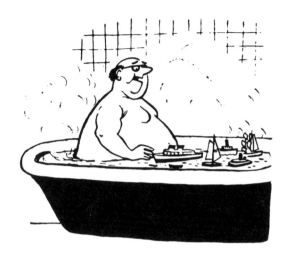

ONCE WEEKLY TAKE THE HOT EPSOM SALTS BATH—
SWEAT-SWEAT-SWEAT!

This hot bath is important to the reducer. It cleanses the pores of the skin.

You must take it once weekly (several times is better).

Directions: Do not start the bath too hot. Get into mildly warm water then gradually add hot water until you reach a toleration point. This should be around 104 degrees (get a bathroom thermometer at the drug store). At this point add one cup of epsom salts. Now remain in the hot water (104 degrees) for at least 10 minutes. The bathroom should be well-heated at this point so that when you drain the water from the tub you can remain the tub and sweat. If the hot bath is taken properly you should have at least 20 miuntes to half an hour sweat. Then shower yourself with cold water and give yourself a good rub down with a coarse towel.

During the time you are in the water, drink at least a pint of warm water and the juice of lemon and a fourth teaspoon of honey.

The filtering action of the kidneys, so important to the removal of toxins from the body, is now augmented by this cleaning sweat. The 96 million pores of your skin now help rid the body of dangerous toxins.

This bath relieves the kidneys of a great deal of hard work.

It is another way to speed the reduction of excess weight.

Strong, smooth, velvety-like skin ... with a healthy pink glow ... firm .. strong and solid. Your muscles will have a certain firmness that will make you proud of them. You will lose fat fast! Fat does not like a pounding healthy circulation just as it doesn't like exercise. Buck up your courage and get into that cold water bath ... you can thank me for the suggestion. So turn on the cold water and have fun!

THESE METHODS ARE FOR BOTH MEN AND WOMEN

My program for Internal Physical Fitness applies equally to men and women. In fact, in some respects the message of this book applies even more strongly to women than it does to men.

Women, as a rule, are more conscious of their physical beings than men are. They are more sensitive to the ageing process, and naturally want to hold on to their youthful beauty and vitality, and retain a good figure and a clear, fresh youthful and attractive complexion. For this reason, they will go to greater efforts to help themselves than most men will.

But in this country, women are very poorly educated in the scientific facts about physical fitness and how to obtain natural beauty from within! They are brain-washed by advertising and publicity urging them to dye their hair, spend hours upon hours in beauty parlors getting beauty treatments, etc . . . all of this to frantically try to remain youthful and beautiful! They are made to believe that beauty and attractiveness come from the outside in. The more creams and lotions they put on their faces, the prettier they will be. Now, cosmetics are sometimes necessary for helping keep the skin clean and moisturized, but creams are not the full answer to the way to keep youthful looking. Cosmetics have their rightful place in a beauty program. But, good natural diet and exercise are what I call "Internal Cosmetics." No vibrating machine can tighten the facial mucles like exercise which will remove ugly fat and fat spots.

For over 60 years I have been Diet Advisor and Physical Conditioner to some of the highest paid movie stars, T.V. stars and actresses in Hollywood. I try to explain to these women that youthful vigor and beauty, good complexion, and a trim but vigorous body can come only from the inside. It is a combination of good natural diet, exercise and a program of deep breathing that will make them beautiful and keep them youthful for many, many years.

Some women shy away from physical fitness programs with the wrong psychological attitude that there is something unfeminine about vigorous exercising of the muscles. I want to impress on every woman the fact that there is absolutely no adequate substitute for planned exercise, walking in the fresh air, swimming and running, no matter what the glamour advertisements may say.

"Men do not die, they KILL themselves."
—Seneca, Roman Philosopher

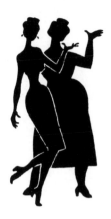

HERE IS THE NATURAL WAY TO REDUCE
IN A NUTSHELL

I personally believe that which is not simple and understandable is humbug. I believe that nature intended us to be of normal weight. We humans are the only beings living on the face of the earth who are of different sizes and shapes. Animals and birds, living a Natural Life, are always of a uniform size. Just look at the fish of the sea. They run normal to size according to their species. This also holds true for the animal and bird kingdoms. But we who are God's highest creation, are of many assorted sizes—fat, skinny, broad, tall and short.

LIPOSUCTION – This new fat removal operation is where an incision is made and the fat is literally sucked out of the body by a little vacuum machine. This does have some drawbacks that could be serious! One is the rupturing of blood vessels and internal bleeding that comes most often with liposuction. However carefully the operation is performed, it still has some dangers! So caution! I saw a young woman who 7 days after she had liposuction had legs that were all black, blue and red with broken veins! I was shocked into thinking if everyone had seen this – no one would ever have this operation! I prefer you monitor your own food intake and step up your daily exercise, for this has no complications and no medical bills!

– Patricia Bragg

Massage brings new changes to the body in many various forms: Unclogging of the body forces and machinery, promotes more circulation flowing, which brings more healing, new feelings and smoother muscular patterns that will in general bring you more vital health! Our inner and outer problems often hit us in the "gut" and muscles, and massage helps in this overall health picture.

It is your birthright to be normal. And you can restore yourself to the human you were supposed to be by following this Natural Way of Reducing. You are fat and over-weight because you ate too much and exercised too little. Now you are going to reverse this situation. You are not going to eat more than your body can manage and you are going to fast, diet and exercise these unwanted pounds away.

First force your Mind to take full command of your body. All commands come from your mind. The body must obey that which your mind commands. You are no longer going to let your base, primitive appetites control you. Always remember that FLESH IS DUMB. And you must NOT be controlled by stupid flesh. The moment your mind is in command you will start to reduce and rebuild the body you desire.

Your fasting program of two 24 hour periods weekly will melt away the fat rapidly. Your non-stimulating diet consisting of a preponderance of raw and cooked non-starchy vegetables will help to mold your body back to its original lines.

Then following your exercise and activity program, you will tone your muscles so they will become strong and supple. As the fat leaves the body, the chest will be free of its burden of fat and you will breathe with ease. You will no longer huff and puff.

Fat, as you know already, smothers the over-weight person. I watch fat people fighting day after day to get enough air into their lungs to survive. It's really pitiful to see these people struggle to get enough air in their lungs to stay alive. The heart and brain need oxygen and the fat person just does not get enough oxygen to the heart and brain. This alone should make an over-weight person want to return to his normal weight. Life is a miserable existence when you have to struggle to get air into your body. So as you shed the excess sick, flabby flesh the lungs will get more air and you will feel alive again. Life is meant to be a joy; but the fat person who has to fight for each breath of air is in a bad way. The fat person's life is always tediously balanced on a razor sharp fence.

Now that no longer has to be the situation. This little book contains all the information you need in order to live the Natural Way of life, to be the slim and trim person you were meant to be.

In my 60 years of working with over-weight people, I have seen thousands win the battle against fat and bloom into fine, healthy persons who now enjoy life with their healthy bodies of normal weight. What joy it is to have a normal body! But you must remember that most fat people must concentrate the rest of their lives on retaining their normal weight through this program. You cannot be lax at any time. Your mind must always be in full command of your body.

CIGARETTES AND OVER-WEIGHT

I often hear people say, "SINCE I GAVE UP CIGAR-ETTES I HAVE GAINED WEIGHT." Of course you did. Cigarettes are one of the most deadly habits a person can have. It's an out-and-out killer. I do not have the space in this small book to tell you of all the dangers involved in using that vile weed. It disturbs the digestion, for one thing, so when you give up the habit, the body makes a violent effort to adjust itself. When the cigarette smoker was smoking he suffered from many deficiencies, particularly of vitamin C, which is the cement of the body. When cigarettes are given up, the body is able to take in and digest more foods with vitamin C and all the other vitamins, minerals and nutrients that the cigarettes had deprived the body of.

The person who gives up the deadly cigarette habit can control his weight with this Natural System of Reducing.

I have taken many men and women off the deadly cigarette habit and put them on this Natural Way of Reducing and they have always lost weight.

Only one-third of smokers gain weight when they give up cigarettes. About as many actually end up losing weight by combining a fitness program with their efforts to quit.

The tobacco industry is the largest advertiser in the print media and on billboards. Its total advertising budget adds up to about $40 for every smoker in the U.S.

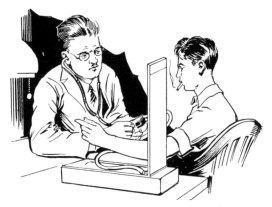

Cigarette smoking always causes a rise in blood pressure.

A WORD OF ADVICE TO THE
CIGARETTE SMOKER

I do not believe I can tell you any more than you have read about the dangers of smoking. You know that when you smoke you are committing suicide. Every smoker whom I knew 50 years ago is now DEAD. I will bury every cigarette smoker I know today. I tell them so.

For your health's sake, for the sake of your life, GIVE UP THIS KILLING HABIT. I believe if you will go on this program it will help you banish the cigarette habit forever. As you fast and the toxic poisons leave your body, your cigarettes will begin to taste putrid. Many of my reducing students have gone on the Natural Way of Reducing and in a few weeks of fasting and purification of the body, they just couldn't smoke any more. So if you are over-weight and smoke you are going to do two good things for yourself at once. You are going to lose the excess weight and you are going to defeat the cigarette habit. A double victory for *YOU*.

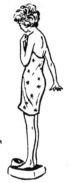

BE PATIENT, THE NATURAL WAY OF REDUCING IS SLOW BUT SURE

You must realize that it has taken you time to gain your excess weight, and it is going to take time to get that weight off in order to firm, trim and slim your body. I am not going to give you any wild promises about how quickly you are going to lose all your excess weight. As you lose weight through the Natural System you want to firm and tone your skin and muscles as you go along. I have seen these "MIRA-CLE" reducing diets. Yes, they took off the weight fast but how did the person look afterward? AWFUL! The loose skin simply hung in a limp fashion on the body frame. The reducer looked prematurely old and haggard. What was left of the flesh was weak, flabby and sick.

This Natural Way of Reducing is one that works with nature and restores the flesh back to its youthful looking condition again.

So do not be impatient. If you will watch your bathroom chart and watch your weight and measurements you will plainly see that you are slimming, trimming and firming again. You see, when you have attained your normal weight I want you to be proud, mighty proud, of your achievement.

HEALTHY HEART HABIT: The king of exercise is brisk walking with arms swinging saying affirmations... "Health, Joy, Peace, Love, Vitality" with every step. Your arms and legs are your 4 powerful health pumps, with your heart the No. 1 pump! With walking you discover the beauty of Nature and it awakens and softens your mind, soul, and life. Your problems and excess weight melt away. You see the changes of Mother Nature and her seasons of new growth, sweet smells after a refreshing, cleansing rain...to the mating, singing bird calls. It's amazing how you can recharge your body, mind and soften your heart with nature walking and giving thanks for all your blessings! No excuses—start your walking program today! —*Patricia Bragg*

70

You are no longer fat. The Natural Way will not only reduce you but it also let you emerge from this program a healthy, vital, ageless person. You will reach a state called AGELESS-NESS.

Once again you will be proud and happy with your body. No longer will you be a frustrated person. No longer will you be ashamed of your body. You will look good with or without clothes. You will have an energetic body. Your body, regardless of your age, will be youthful looking. And by following your Natural Way of living you can add many years to your life. You will now be an active person physically; you will be able to walk for miles, dance for hours, swim, work and thrill in the joy of living.

We have buried the over-weight person you were. You are new, all new. Health is truly wealth. Your body is your treasure. You hold this priceless possession in the palm of your hands.

Be jealous of your health. Let nothing or no one turn you away from your joyous new life. Let the fat weaklings indulge themselves. You will live to see them sicken and die long before their time.

When you are tempted to over-eat or eat fattening food, summon your Mind-Power to give battle to this temptation. We are all human and we *DO* weaken. Don't condemn yourself but go on a fast for several days to compensate for your indiscretion.

Only 20% of American's have some form of regular exercise! This is causing poor health and mounting cardiovascular disease. A regular exercise program is important for heart health — Start your daily exercise program today.

Buy the best in walking and athletic shoes. Be sure they fit perfect and the heels are well padded. Your heels bear 60% of your weight.

NOW ABOUT THOSE SEVEN TO TEN DAY FASTS

I purposely waited until the end of the book to tell you about this part of the Natural Way of Reducing. I wanted you to get an overall picture of the program.

Now you are ready to accomplish the core of this program. But first let me tell you about myself. I am a person who gains weight easily. Ever since I regained my health from tuberculosis years ago I have always had to keep a careful check on my weight.

I am 5 feet eight inches tall, so therefore my ideal weight is 165 pounds, but I keep my weight under 160 pounds. Four times a year, I go on a 7 to 10 day fast. I stop eating and use nothing but water to drink. I always break my fast in the same manner. After I have finished seven days of fasting, on the evening of that seventh day, I eat a dish of stewed fresh tomatoes which have been peeled. On the morning of the eighth day I have, for my first meal, a dish of salad consisting of chopped cabbage, shredded carrots and chopped celery.

I use a small amount of dressing made of lemon juice or pure natural apple cider vinegar and oil. I eat my fill of the salad, then I have a dish of cooked greens and tomatoes. You can select any greens available—spinach, mustard greens, kale, beet tops or turnip tops. I have this for the first meal after the long fast and I repeat this same meal later on in the day. The next day I return to my regular diet. My diet is about the same as I have given you.

You must keep constantly in mind that raw salads and cooked non-starch vegetables with proteins of your choice are going to help you melt fat away. And the fasting is gradually going to help you melt away those spots of hidden fat.

Hidden fat will collect in various parts of the body, particularly on the abdomen. Our non-stimulating diet will melt most of the fat from the abdomen, but it takes a 7 to 10 day fast to really eliminate that locked-in fat.

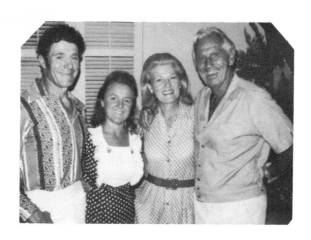

Jack LaLanne, Patricia Bragg, Elaine LaLanne & Paul Bragg

Jack says, "Bragg saved my life at age 15 when I attended the Bragg Health & Fitness Crusade in Oakland, California." From that day on Jack has lived the health life & has inspired millions to Health & Fitness.

Woman will carry the locked-in fat on their breasts, hips, on the upper back, on the upper arms, inside thighs, stomach and back of the knees. It is the cleansing and purifying fast that burns off locked-in fat areas. Nothing else works as well as fasting along with daily exercise, deep breathing and living the Bragg Healthy Lifestyle.

In men the locked-in fat will cling to the chin, cheeks, jaws, chest, stomach and particularly the hips and thighs.

A few years ago a man and wife came to me. Both were more than 50 pounds over-weight. They were not only over-weight, this weight was mostly hard, locked-in fat on the parts of the body that I have just mentioned. They had had a complete physical examination and were told that their health was in serious condition due to their over-weight. Remember, fat people are most always filled with ailments.

Massage helps in soothing, releasing and making you aware of the body. The trained "touch-skilled" therapist using their hands and fingers as a diagnostic tool can feel the locked-in areas. Often toxic crystals and toxic wastes get locked up in knotted muscles, connective tissues and sore, previous injured areas. A good therapist has in their hands the ability to help the body flush out these toxins which will help restore more health to the tissues by releasing these toxins! Remember the body is self-repairing and self-healing when given the opportunity. Massages are important cleansing, healing health aids!

73

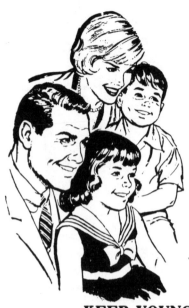

LIFE'S GREATEST TREASURE IS RADIANT HEALTH

"There is no substitute for Health. Those who possess it are richer than kings."

KEEP YOUNG BIOLOGICALLY
WITH EXERCISE AND GOOD NUTRITION

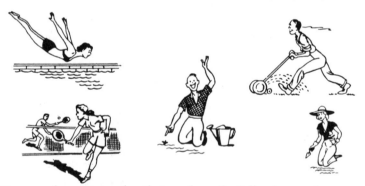

You can always remember that you have the following good reasons for sticking to your health program:

- The ironclad laws of Nature.
- Your common sense which tells you that you are doing right.
- Your aim to make your health better and your life longer.
- Your resolve to prevent illness so that you may enjoy life.
- By making an art of life, you will be young at any age.
- You will retain your faculties and be hale, hearty, active and useful far beyond the ordinary length of days, and you will also possess superior mental and physical powers.

These people were simply two over-fed butterballs. They had tried "crash" diet; diets which promised easy reduction. But here they were; fat and sick. They saw the hand-writing on the wall, they knew something tragic was about to happen if they did not do something immediately.

Their condition was so serious that I started them both on a seven day fast. This imposed a hardship on these two sick people but something drastic had to be done. Their lives were hanging by a thin thread.

Believe it or not, they did remarkably well on this seven day fast. Their fat toxic bodies reacted well to the physiological housecleaning produced by the fast. Their stomachs shrank and they did not demand the quantity of food that they had been accustomed to eating. The remarkable part of the fast was that the locked-in fat on their bodies began to melt away. Those first seven days did the trick, and from then on they steadily lost pounds and inches off their bodies.

Today, two years later, they are of normal weight and have shed from their bodies all the locked-in fat which they carried when they first came to me for reduction.

The reduction was perfect and I was delighted that they lost so much weight. But their physical condition was what fascinated me the most. Recently, they had a complete physical examination and they received a clean slate. The doctors could find nothing wrong with them; their hearts, pulse rates, blood pressures, urine and everything else checked out perfectly.

In the two years that they were under my personal supervision they fasted faithfully two 24 hour periods weekly, and four times a year I had them fast from seven to ten days. This is exactly how the Natural Way of Reducing works, slow but sure. These people did not have a lot of loose, flabby overstretched skin on their bodies after they had attained their normal weight. The skin and muscle tone of their bodies are splendid. Naturally, they have been faithful with their exercise program and their cold baths and friction rubs with a coarse towel.

So please let me repeat: fasting is absolutely the *only* way to melt away locked-in fat. I know this to be true because I have studied reducing methods all over the world, and I have seen people reduced by various methods, but when I checked these people the deposits of locked-in fat still remained and; their reducing had left them with loose, hanging flesh all over their body.

It boils down to this, if you are really serious about reducing your weight, this locked-in fat must be considered first as the most dangerous fat on your body.

Now we have visible locked-in fat that we can see but what about the invisible fat that is smothering your heart? That locked-in fat which is damaging your liver, kidneys and other vital organs of the body.

As I have told you, I am vitally interested in your personal appearance. I want you to look good dressed or undressed. I look upon fat as a deadly killer. Fat people are subject to many, many dangerous diseases and fat people are short-lived. So when you go on a fast you are actually saving your own life. Fasting is the natural way to melt fat away and flush out the deadly toxic poisons that are killing you.

At the Health Resort which I conducted in California for 25 years, I had hundreds of fat people who desired to be reduced. Some of them were 200 pounds or more over-weight. They were examined by doctors carefully before they went on the Natural Way of Reducing program and after they had been reduced to their normal weight. In every instance, they not only reduced but they gained a new health. Remember, when you get rid of fat you're getting rid of sick flesh which is highly toxic. Every pound of excess fat you carry on your body is sick and toxic, and if you don't get it off and get it off soon, you are in for serious troubles.

It Takes a positive-minded person to take control of their body. Any butterball can let the body rule them. Fasting is the greatest of all disciplines. Until you can fast, *YOU* are not the master of your body . . . any fat person can go on reducing diets. That is still eating. Fasting is when you stop eating, and drink only distilled water.

I wish there were easy methods for reducing. The Natural Way to Reduce is therapeutic reducing. It flushes toxic poisons out of the body as it reduces. No other system of reducing ever attempts this. I have often seen people reduce, but they had not lost their toxic poisons, and were sick reduced people. In reducing, they had demineralized and devitaminized themselves.

OBESE PEOPLE HAVE SICK LIVERS

I know from extensive and lengthy experience in reducing thousands of people, that obese people have sick livers. The liver is the #1 chemical laboratory in the body as well as its most important detoxifier. It is so vital to us that we can only live a few hours without it. Obese people have exhausted, sick livers. So just going on a reducing diet is not going to restore an exhausted liver. Only by water and juice fasting, which gives the liver a physiological rest and cleansing. The liver is the body's main organ of detoxification. It is the strainer through which is poured all fluids before they enter the general circulatory system. As long as the liver is doing its vital work of purification, the bloodstream remains healthy and clean. When it becomes exhausted, as it does when people are carrying excess poisons in the form of fat, the vile toxins enter the circulation and cause violent destruction to the vital organs of the body and then the final stage . . . *death!*

Dick Gregory, Famous Comedian and Author, weighed 320 pounds and his inspiration to health and fitness was the Bragg "Miracle of Fasting" Book. He traded his bad habits — dead, processed foods, drinking, drugs, smoking, etc. for healthy habits! He's now a trim 150 pounds, been in eight Boston Marathons and is now busy guiding others to reduce and enjoy healthy lifestyle living!

Ten Two Letter Words To Live By;
If It Is To Be . . . It Is Up To Me!

When the liver is exhausted, the vicious toxic poisons back up into other parts of the body—the same as when a toilet overflows. Serious trouble is near at hand.

Just going on a reducing diet is not going to correct an exhausted liver. Fasting is the only method by which you will be able to restore the liver back to its original, efficient power. Fasting restores this efficient full activity to not only the liver, but to the kidneys as well, which in turn helps you to enjoy a superior state of health and well-being.

The body is a self-healing and self-repairing instrument. Your body is constantly fighting a biological battle for its survival. When you fast, you help it with that survival. If you will work with the recuperative forces within your body you can attain normal weight and with it, a healthy body. Maintaining normal weight and health is not something bestowed on you by beneficent nature at birth; it is achieved and maintained only by active participation in the well-defined laws of healthful living. You have excess fat because you are not living by Natural Law.

Healthful living is a way of life. The world is full of fat, sick people who refuse to live by Nature's Master Plan of Living.

Instead of enjoying glowing health and normal weight which is our birthright, most people live haphazard lives. These are the people who fill the doctor's offices crying out for help; these are the people who are on their bed of pain in the hospitals and the ones in wheel-chairs and the ones for whom life is snuffed-out long before their time.

ADMIT YOUR GUILT—THEN DO SOMETHING ABOUT IT

Most people want to blame their over-weight condition on anything but themselves. You are over-weight because you do not know how to live by Nature's Master Plan.

The book you are now reading gives you the blue-print for living by Nature's Plan. Your over-weight, your pain, your tormenting misery and illness result from your unnatural way of eating and living. You are fat and suffering because you are filled with vile toxic wastes caused by your poorly selected food, filled with artificial flavorings, preservatives, synthetics, over-processed ingredients; too much stimulating food, and too few Natural minerals from vegetables and fruit.

Your excess fat is simply stored up poisons that your over-worked body cannot get rid of. Fat is the sickest of the sick flesh; it is ugly and it is burdensome. If you have one ounce of courage and determination in you, start this Natural Way of Reducing TODAY . . . not tomorrow. Tomorrow may be too late.

Any weakling can find excuses and alibis for not starting this program. They belong to the legion of the doomed.

But the person with a spark of real spunk will say "I will start this moment on the Natural Way to Reduce." I *dare* you to be a positive person and follow this program! I *challenge* you to make this fight against the fat that is dragging you down to illness and an early grave!

You can if you are really in dead earnest about reducing to your normal weight and then maintaining it.

Other students of mine have done it and they are the happiest people on earth. Now, it is your turn to fight your battle against deadly, sick, ugly slobby fat. Here are the do-it-yourself tools to create in yourself the person you want to be. There is nothing to stop you except your own hesitant, negative self. Your fat is going to kill you or you are going to kill it. You have a brain. The Creator gave you this priceless treasure to use for your survival. You can use your brain or your stomach. The brain is a tool God gave in order for you to rule over your flesh and thereby help to preserve your life. The stomach is just dumb flesh, you can put anything you want in it. You can over-load it—abuse it. Brain or stomach: who will win? Brain! Good, I knew that would be your decision. Now go to it. Don't let any negative thoughts stop you. Don't let any of your ignorant, weak-willed relatives and friends drag you down to their level.

YOU are doing the positive thinking and the positive action from this moment on. Good-bye fat. YOU are on the road to a slim, trim, youthful and healthy body. From this moment on "THINK THIN." Keep saying to yourself, "I will be thin." For as he thinketh in his heart so is he (Prov. 23:7). And as *YOU* think in *YOUR* heart so *YOU* WILL BE.

THINK TRIM, FIT AND HEALTHY!!!

Start today on your Natural Reducing Program. Refuse to let fat be your master.

Patricia Bragg   *Paul C. Bragg*

Healthy Mind Habit: Wake up and say – "Today I am going to be happier, healthier and wiser in my daily living, as I am the "captain" of my life and am going to steer it for 100% healthy living!" Fact – Happy people look younger and have fewer health problems! — Patricia Bragg

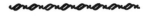

"Why not look for the best – the best in others, the best in ourselves, the best in all life situations? He who looks for the best knows the worst is there but refuses to be discouraged by it. Though temporarily defeated, dismayed, he smiles and tries again. If you look for the best, life will become pleasant for you and everyone around you."

— *REV. Paul S. Osumi*

DESIRABLE WEIGHTS

M E N
WEIGHT IN POUNDS

HEIGHT 1" heels	Small Frame	Medium Frame	Large Frame
5 ft. 2 in.	112-120	118-129	129-141
5 ft. 3 in.	115-123	121-133	129-144
5 ft. 4 in.	118-126	124-136	132-148
5 ft. 5 in.	121-129	127-139	135-152
5 ft. 6 in.	124-133	130-143	138-156
5 ft. 7 in.	128-137	134-147	142-161
5 ft. 8 in.	132-141	138-152	147-166
5 ft. 9 in.	136-145	142-156	151-170
5 ft. 10 in.	140-150	146-160	155-174
5 ft. 11 in.	144-154	150-165	159-179
6 ft.	148-158	154-170	164-184
6 ft. 1 in.	152-162	158-175	168-189
6 ft. 2 in.	156-167	162-180	173-194
6 ft. 3 in.	160-171	167-185	178-199
6 ft. 4 in.	164-175	172-190	182-204

W O M E N
WEIGHT IN POUNDS

HEIGHT 2" heels	Frame Small	Frame Medium	Frame Large
4 ft. 10 in.	92- 98	96-107	104-119
4 ft. 11 in.	94-101	98-110	106-122
5 ft.	96-104	101-113	109-125
5 ft. 1 in.	99-107	104-116	112-128
5 ft. 2 in.	102-110	107-119	115-131
5 ft. 3 in.	105-113	110-122	118-134
5 ft. 4 in.	108-116	113-126	121-138
5 ft. 5 in.	111-119	116-130	125-142
5 ft. 6 in.	114-123	120-135	129-146
5 ft. 7 in.	118-127	124-139	133-150
5 ft. 8 in.	122-131	128-143	137-154
5 ft. 9 in.	126-135	132-147	141-158
5 ft. 10 in.	130-140	136-151	145-163
5 ft. 11 in.	134-144	140-155	149-168
6 ft.	138-148	144-159	153-173

Drink Health the Live, Raw Juice Way, For Reducing

ALL OVER THE United States we hear about "cocktail hours" where beautifully colored alcoholic creations are used to produce new thrills, stimulate jaded appetites and bolster failing spirits.

We have a new kind of "cocktail," thanks to my dad Paul C. Bragg. It is not made of whisky, gin, rum or other alcoholic substance. There isn't a pickled cherry to be found in one of them. These live, recharging juices are made from fresh, organically grown vegetables and ripe fruits — the very life-blood of the plant – to boost your energy and immune levels. Dad imported the first hand juicers from Europe and with the Bragg Crusades introduced juice therapy across America. There is no liquor on the face of the earth so satisfying as the fresh live juice cocktail. Not only is it delicious but there is something more — the satisfaction and nourishment of the billions of cells that make up your body. When people take to the health cocktail habit, they are putting the plants' liquid life into their bodies to supercharge their health!

When we consider that fruits and vegetables have been grown naturally by solar energy (sunshine), they contain all of the elements that the sun and earth have buried deep into their fibrous cells, they are live cell foods. Juicing is a convenient and inexpensive method of obtaining the most concentrated form of nutrition available from the whole plant foods.

Select & Prepare Organic Foods for Juicing Whenever Possible ... because commercial produce can contain deadly pesticides and petrochemical fertilizers. Yearly over 2.6 billion pounds of pesticides are dumped on American food crops. Choose deep-colored, ripe, firm fruits and fresh healthy vegetables. Use both the leaves and stems as well as the body of the vegetable. They yield an abundance of organic minerals. The tops of the carrots, for instance, contain phosphorus.

Raw, live fruit and vegetable juices can be purchased fresh from most Health Food Stores or prepared at home with one of the new wonderful juicers on the market. These health juices can be used full strength or diluted with distilled water on fasting days.

"Every healthy horse has some gas!" stated American farmers. When people eat healthy, natural plant fiber foods (fresh fruits, vegetables, and whole-grains), they are cleaning, purifying and recharging their body machinery. Occasionally some gentle cleansing combustion (gas) will occur. There is a new enzyme product that helps with this (especially with beans) called Beano.

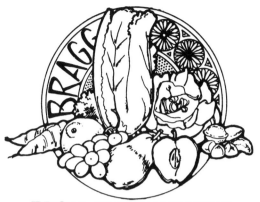

FROM THE AUTHORS

This book was written for YOU. It can be your passport to the Good Life. We Professional Nutritionists join hands in one common objective — a high standard of health for all and many added years to your life. Scientific Nutrition points the way — Nature's Way — the only lasting way to build a body free of degenerative diseases and premature aging. This book teaches you how to work with Nature and not against her. Doctors, dentists, and others who care for the sick, try to repair depleted tissues which too often mend poorly if at all. Many of them praise the spreading of this new scientific message of natural foods and methods for long-lasting health and youth-fulness at any age. To speed the spreading of this tremendous message, this book was written.

Statements in this book are recitals of scientific findings, known facts of physiology, biological therapeutics, and reference to ancient writings as they are found. Paul C. Bragg has been practicing the natural methods of living for over 70 years, with highly beneficial results, knowing they are safe and of great value to others, and his daughter Patricia Bragg works with him to carry on the Health Crusade. They make no claims as to what the methods cited in this book will do for one in any given situation, and assume no obligation because of opinions expressed.

No cure for disease is offered in this book. No foods or diets are of-fered for the treatment or cure of any specific ailment. Nor is it in-tended as, or to be used as, literature for any food product. Paul C. Bragg and Patricia Bragg express their opinions solely as Public Health Educators, Professional Nutritionists and Teachers.

Certain persons considered experts may disagree with one or more statements in this book, as the same relate to various nutritional recommendations. However, any such statements are considered, nevertheless, to be factual, as based upon long-time experience of Paul C. Bragg and Patricia Bragg in the field of human health.

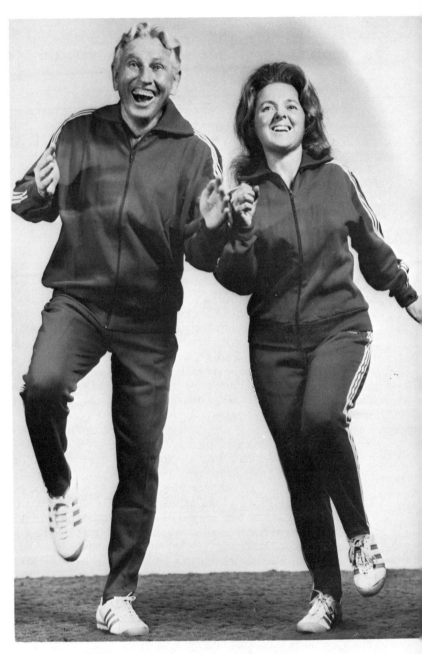

Paul Bragg and daughter Patricia carry out a vigorous
morning exercise program faithfully every day,
and keep in peak physical condition.

PAUL C. BRAGG N.D., Ph.D.

Life Extension Specialist • World Health Crusader
Lecturer and Advisor to Olympic Athletes, Royalty, and Stars
Originator of Health Food Stores - Now World-wide

For almost a Century, Living Proof that his
"Health and Fitness Way of Life" Works Wonders!

Paul C. Bragg is the Father of the Health Movement in America. This dynamic Crusader for worldwide health and fitness is responsible for more "firsts" in the history of Health than any other individual. Here are a few of his incredible pioneering achievements that the world now enjoys:

- Bragg originated, named and opened the first "Health Food Store" in America.
- Bragg Crusades pioneered the first Health Lectures across America, inspiring followers to open health stores in cities across the land and now world-wide.
- Bragg introduced pineapple juice and tomato juice to the American public.
- He was the first to introduce and distribute honey nationwide.
- He introduced Juice Therapy in America by importing the first hand-juicers.
- Bragg pioneered Radio Health Programs from Hollywood three times daily. Paul and Patricia pioneered a Health TV show from Hollywood to spread "Health and Happiness"... the name of the show! It included exercises, health recipes, visual demonstrations, and guest appearances of famous, health-minded people.
- He created the first health foods & products and made them available nation-wide: herb teas, health beverages, seven-grain cereals and crackers, health cosmetics, health candies, vitamins and mineral supplements, wheat germ, digestive enzymes from papaya, herbs & kelp seasonings, amino acids from soybeans. He inspired others to follow and now thousands of health items are available worldwide.
- He opened the first health restaurants and health spas in America.

Crippled by TB as a teenager, Bragg developed his own eating, breathing and exercising program to rebuild his body into an ageless, tireless, painfree citadel of glowing, radiant health. He excelled in running, swimming, biking, progressive weight training, and mountain-climbing. He made an early pledge to God, in return for his renewed health, to spend the rest of his life showing others the road to health... Paul Bragg made good his pledge!

A living legend and beloved counselor to millions, Bragg was the inspiration and personal advisor on diet and fitness to top Olympic Stars from 4-time swimming Gold Medalist Murray Rose to 3-time track Gold Medalist Betty Cuthbert of Australia, his relative Don Bragg (pole-vaulting Gold Medalist), and countless others. Jack LaLanne, "the original TV King of Fitness," says, "Bragg saved my life at age 14 when I attended the Bragg Crusade in Oakland, California." From the earliest days, Bragg was advisor to the greatest Hollywood Stars, and to giants of American Business. J. C. Penney, Del E. Webb, and Conrad Hilton are just a few that he inspired to long, successful, healthy, active lives!

Dr. Bragg changed the lives of millions worldwide in all walks of life... through his Health Crusades, Books, Tapes and Radio, TV and personal appearances.

HEALTH SCIENCE Box 7, Santa Barbara, California 93102 U.S.A.

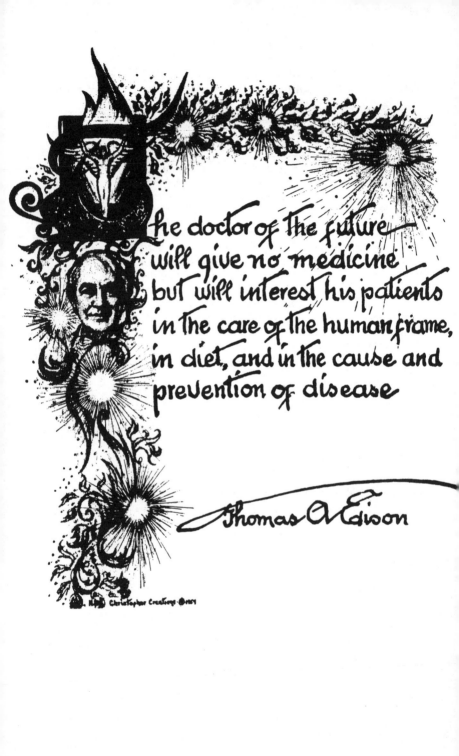

The doctor of the future
will give no medicine
but will interest his patients
in the care of the human frame,
in diet, and in the cause and
prevention of disease

Thomas A. Edison

BRAGG "HOW-TO, SELF HEALTH" BOOKS
Authored by America's First Family of Health
Live Longer – Healthier – Stronger Self-Improvement Library

Qty.	Bragg Book Titles Order Form Health Science ISBN 0-87790	Price	Total $
____	**Vegetarian** Gourmet Health **Recipes** (no salt, no sugar, yet delicious)	7.95	•
____	Bragg's Complete **Gourmet Recipes** for Vital Health—448 pages	8.95	•
____	The **Miracle of Fasting** (Bragg Bible of Health for physical rejuvenation)	6.95	•
____	Bragg **Health & Fitness Manual** for All Ages—Swim-Bike-Run A Must for Athletes, Triathletes & Would-Be-Athletes—600 pages	*16.95	•
____	Build Powerful **Nerve Force** (reduce stress, fear, anger, worry)	5.95	•
____	Keep Your **Heart** & Cardio-Vascular System Healthy & Fit at Any Age	5.95	•
____	The Natural Way to **Reduce** (lose 10 pounds in 10 days)	5.95	•
____	The Shocking Truth About **Water** (learn safest water to drink & why)	5.95	•
____	Your Health and Your **Hair**, Nature's Way to Beautiful Hair (easy-to-do method) .	5.95	•
____	**Healthful Eating** Without Confusion (removes doubt & questions)	5.95	•
____	Salt-Free Raw **Sauerkraut Recipes** (learn to make your own)	2.95	•
____	Nature's Healing System to Improve **Eyesight** in 90 days (foods, exercises, etc.)	5.95	•
____	Super Brain **Breathing** for Super Health & High Energy (can double your energy)	3.95	•
____	Building Strong **Feet** — Complete Program	5.95	•
____	**Toxicless Diet**-Purification & Healing System (Stay Ageless Program)	3.95	•
____	Powerful Health Uses of **Apple Cider Vinegar** (how to live active to 120)	3.95	•
____	**Fitness/Spine Motion** – For More Flexible, Pain-free Back	3.95	•
____	Building **Health & Youthfulness**	1.75	•
____	**Nature's Way** to Health (simple method for long, healthy life)	3.95	•
____	The Philosophy of **Super Health**	1.75	•
____	**South Sea Abdomen Culture** for Perfect Elimination & Trim Waist	1.75	•

| **Total Copies** | Prices subject to change without notice. | **TOTAL BOOKS** | $ | • |

Shipping: Please add $1.50 for first book and 75¢ each additional or $3.00 each for airmail

* Add $3.00 shipping for each Bragg Fitness Manual
U.S. retail book orders over $20 add $3.00 only

Shipping & Handling	
Ca. Residents add sales tax	•
TOTAL ENCLOSED $	•

Please Specify:

☐ Check ☐ Money Order ☐ Cash ☐ Credit Card

Please U.S. funds only

Charge My Order To: ☐ Visa ☐ MasterCard   month   year

Credit Card Number: __ __ __ __ — __ __ __ __ — __ __ __ __ — __ __ __ __   Card Expires: ____ | ____

MasterCard *VISA* Signature: _____

CREDIT CARD CUSTOMERS ONLY USE OUR FAST ORDER SERVICE: (800)-446-1990

In a hurry? Call (805) 968-1020. We can accept MasterCard or VISA phone orders only. Please prepare your order using this order form. It will speed your call & serve as your order record. Hours: 9 to 4pm Pacific Time, Monday to Thursday ... or you can fax your order: **FAX (805) 968-1001**.

Mail to: HEALTH SCIENCE, Box 7, Santa Barbara, CA 93102 U.S.A.
Please Print or Type – Be sure to give street & house number to facilitate delivery

BOF-9201

Name _____

Address _____ Apt. No. _____

City _____ State _____

Phone ( ) _____   Zip __ __ __ __ __

Order your Bragg Health Books Today – For a Healthier Tomorrow!

SEND FOR IMPORTANT FREE HEALTH BULLETINS

Let Patricia Bragg send you, your relatives and friends the latest
News Bulletins on Health and Nutrition Discoveries. These are
sent periodically. Please enclose two stamps for each U.S.A.
name listed. Foreign listings send international postal reply
coupons. Please print or type addresses, thank you.

HEALTH SCIENCE Box 7, Santa Barbara, California 93102 U.S.A.

●

Name

_____ ( ) _____
Address   Phone

City   State   Zip Code

●

Name

_____ ( ) _____
Address   Phone

City   State   Zip Code

●

Name

_____ ( ) _____
Address   Phone

City   State   Zip Code

●

Name

_____ ( ) _____
Address   Phone

City   State   Zip Code

●

Name

_____ ( ) _____
Address   Phone

City   State   Zip Code

BRAGG ALL NATURAL LIQUID AMINOS
Order Form

Delicious, Healthy Alternative to Tamari-Soy Sauce

BRAGG LIQUID AMINOS — Nutrition you need...taste you will love...a family favorite for over 75 years. A delicious source of nutritious life-renewing protein from soybeans only. Add to or spray over casseroles, soups, sauces, gravies, potatoes, popcorn, and vegetables. An ideal "pick-me-up" broth at work, home or the gym. Gourmet health replacement for Tamari & Soy Sauce. Start today and add more Amino Acids for healthy living to your daily diet — the easy BRAGG LIQUID AMINOS Way!

DASH or SPRAY for NEW TASTE DELIGHTS! PROVEN & ENJOYED BY MILLIONS.

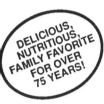

DELICIOUS, NUTRITIOUS, FAMILY FAVORITE FOR OVER 75 YEARS!

Dash of Bragg Aminos Brings New Taste Delights to Season:		Pure Soybeans and Pure Water Only
■ Salads ■ Dressings ■ Soups		■ No Added Sodium
■ Vegies ■ Rice/Beans ■ Tofu		■ No Coloring Agents
■ Tempeh ■ Wok foods ■ Stir-frys		■ No Preservatives
■ Casseroles & Potatoes ■ Meats		■ Not Fermented
■ Poultry ■ Fish ■ Popcorn		■ No Chemicals
■ Gravies ■ Sauces ■ Macrobiotics		■ No Additives
		■ No MSG

BRAGG LIQUID AMINOS

SIZE	PRICE	SHIPPING	AMT.	TOTAL $
16 oz.	$ 3.95 ea.	Please add $3.00 for 1st bottle/$1.50 for each additional bottle		.
32 oz.	$ 6.45 ea.	Please add $3.90 for 1st bottle/$1.90 for each additional bottle		.
16 oz.	$ 47.40 ea.	Case/12 bottles add $9.00 per case		.
32 oz.	$ 77.40 ea.	Case/12 bottles add $14.00 per case		.

Total Aminos	$
Shipping & Handling	.
Total Enclosed	$.

Please Specify: (U.S. Funds Only)

☐ Check   ☐ Money Order   ☐ Cash   ☐ Credit Card

Charge My Order To: ☐ Visa   ☐ MasterCard

Credit Card
Number: _ _ _ _ _ _ _ _ _ _ _ _ _ _ _ _   Card Expires: ___ | ___   Month Year

MasterCard VISA Signature: _____

CREDIT CARD CUSTOMERS ONLY USE OUR FAST PHONE SERVICE: (800) 446-1990

In a hurry? Call (805) 968-1028. We can accept MasterCard & VISA phone orders only. Please prepare your order using this order form. It will speed your call & serve as your order record. Hours: 9 to 4 pm Pacific Time, Monday to Thursday ... or you can fax your order to: **FAX (805) 968-1001.**

Mail to: **HEALTH SCIENCE, Box 7, Santa Barbara, CA 93102 USA**

Please Print or Type – Be sure to give street & house number to facilitate delivery

A-BOF-9201

Name _____

Address _____   Apt. No. _____

City _____   State _____

(____) _____

Phone   Zip _ _ _ _ _

Bragg Aminos —Taste You Love, Nutrition You Need

PATRICIA BRAGG N.D., Ph.D.
Angel of Health & Healing
Lecturer, Author, Nutritionist, Health Educator & Fitness Advisor to World Leaders, Glamorous Hollywood Stars, Singers, Dancers & Athletes.

Daughter of the world renowned health authority, Paul C. Bragg, Patricia Bragg has won international fame on her own in this field. She conducts Health and Fitness Seminars for Women's, Men's, Youth and Church Groups throughout the world... and promotes Bragg "How-To, Self-Health" Books in Lectures, on Radio and Television Talk Shows throughout the English-speaking world. Consultants to Presidents and Royalty, to the Stars of Stage, Screen and TV and to Champion Athletes, Patricia Bragg and her father are Co-Authors of the Bragg Health Library of Instructive, Inspiring Books that promote a healthy lifestyle for a long, vital, active life!

Patricia herself is the symbol of perpetual youth and super energy. She is a living and sparkling example of her and her father's healthy lifestyle precepts and this she shares world-wide.

A fifth generation Californian on her mother's side, Patricia was reared by the Natural Health Method from infancy. In school, she not only excelled in athletics but also won high honors in her studies and her counseling. She is an accomplished musician and dancer... as well as tennis player, swimmer and mountain climber... and the youngest woman ever to be granted a U.S. Patent. Patricia is a popular gifted Health Teacher and a dynamic, in-demand Talk Show Guest where she spreads simple, easy-to-follow health teachings for everyone.

Man's body is the Temple of the Holy Spirit, and our creator wants us filled with Joy and Health for a long walk with Him for Eternity. The Bragg Crusade of Health and Fitness (3 John 2) has carried her around the world... spreading physical, spiritual, emotional and mental health and joy. Health is our birthright and Patricia teaches how to prevent the destruction of our health from man-made wrong habits of living.

Patricia's been Health Consultant to American Presidents and to the British Royal Family, to Betty Cuthbert, Australia's "Golden Girl" who holds 16 world records and four Olympic gold medals in women's track and to New Zealand's Olympic Track Star Allison Roe. Among those who come to her for advice are some of Hollywood's top stars from Clint Eastwood to the ever youthful singing group The Beach Boys and their families, singing stars of the Metropolitan Opera and top ballet stars. Patricia's message is of world-wide appeal to the people of all ages, nationalities and walks-of-life. Those who follow the Bragg Health Books & attend the Bragg Crusades are living testimonials like Super Athlete, Ageless - Jack LaLanne—at age 14 he went from sickness to health.

Patricia Bragg inspires you to Renew, Rejuvenate & Revitalize your life with the "Bragg Healthy Lifestyle" Seminars and Lectures world-wide. These are life-changing and millions have benefited with a longer, healthier life! She would love to share her Crusade with your organizations, businesses, churches, etc. Also, she is a perfect radio and T.V. talk show guest to spread the message of health and fitness in your area.

Write or call for requests and information:
HEALTH SCIENCE, BOX 7, SANTA BARBARA, CA 93102 1-805-968-1028